Practical Guide to

Medical Student Assessment

Practical Guide to **Medical Student Assessment**

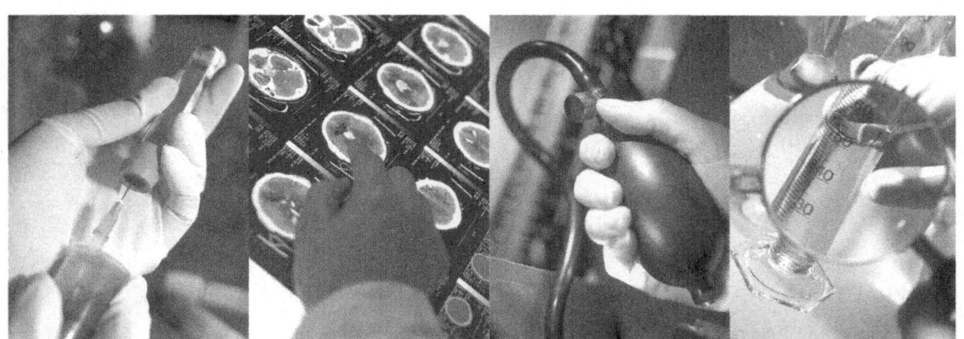

Zubair Amin
Chong Yap Seng
Khoo Hoon Eng

National University of Singapore

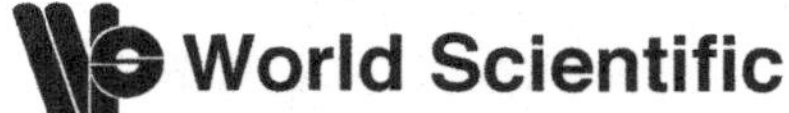

NEW JERSEY • LONDON • SINGAPORE • BEIJING • SHANGHAI • HONG KONG • TAIPEI • CHENNAI

Published by

World Scientific Publishing Co. Pte. Ltd.
5 Toh Tuck Link, Singapore 596224
USA office: 27 Warren Street, Suite 401-402, Hackensack, NJ 07601
UK office: 57 Shelton Street, Covent Garden, London WC2H 9HE

British Library Cataloguing-in-Publication Data
A catalogue record for this book is available from the British Library.

First published 2006
Reprinted 2010

PRACTICAL GUIDE TO MEDICAL STUDENT ASSESSMENT

ISBN-13 978-981-256-808-3
ISBN-10 981-256-808-5

Typeset by Stallion Press
Email: enquiries@stallionpress.com

Printed in Singapore

For Professor Matthew Gwee
Mentor, Teacher, and Educator Extraordinaire

Foreword

Assessment of medical students is one of the ways of affirming our obligation to society and to the public at large. Through assessment we can ensure that our future doctors have acquired the necessary competency to work as physicians and are capable of meeting the demands of society's healthcare needs.

The competent delivery of healthcare requires not just knowledge and technical skills, but must include other qualities such as communication, counselling, interdisciplinary care, and evidence- and system-based care. Therefore, our assessment system needs to be comprehensive and robust enough to assess these attributes along with testing for essential knowledge and skills. It is also imperative that the assessment system meets the requisite criteria of a good assessment by addressing the issues of validity, reliability, fairness and transparency.

As medical teachers, it is our professional responsibility to update ourselves on best practices and best evidence in assessment and to make a conscious educated effort in implementing them.

The success of these endeavours depends on easy and concise information on the various methods of assessment. Three of my colleagues have taken the initiative to write this very practical and much needed guide on assessment. This guide should give medical teachers the necessary knowledge and confidence to design valid, reliable, fair and transparent assessment for their students.

Professor John Wong
Dean, Yong Loo Lin School of Medicine
National University of Singapore
Singapore
January 2006

Acknowledgement

We thank our fellow members of the Medical Education Unit and Education Task Force, Yong Loo Lin School of Medicine, National University of Singapore, Drs Matthew Gwee, Koh Dow Rhoon, Tan Chay Hoon, Goh Poh Sun, and Lau Tang Ching who first reviewed the Guide. We also gratefully acknowledge the comments and suggestions made by the various heads of the departments in the Yong Loo Lin School of Medicine. Our special thanks to Ms Linda Lim, from the Publication Support Unit, National University Hospital and National University of Singapore, for editing the draft.

The views expressed here are those of the authors only and do not necessarily reflect the official position of the Medical Education Unit, Yong Loo Lin School of Medicine or other bodies.

Acknowledgement

About the Authors

Dr Zubair Amin is a pediatrician and medical educator. He was trained in Pediatrics in the University of Illinois at Chicago. He has a Master in Health Profession Education (MHPE) from the same university. His interests and expertise are in assessment, staff development and international medical education.

Dr Chong Yap Seng is an obstetrician and educational leader. He is a graduate from National University of Singapore. He is deeply involved in undergraduate and postgraduate education, faculty training, assessment and scientific writing. He is the Head of Medical Education Unit, Yong Loo Lin School of Medicine, National University of Singapore.

Dr Khoo Hoon Eng is Associate Professor in the Department of Biochemistry, Yong Loo Lin School of Medicine, National University of Singapore. She has a BA from Smith College, USA, PhD from University of London and Diploma in Medical Education from University of Dundee, UK. Her interests are in problem based learning, faculty training, and assessment.

About the Authors

About this Guide

The purpose of this Guide is to provide a simple, practical reference to commonly raised questions about assessment instruments.

In preparing this Guide we have taken into consideration issues that are, in our collective opinion, pertinent to the medical, nursing, and para-medical faculty. Therefore, instead of pursuing the rather impossible goal of being all-inclusive, we have focused on selected assessment instruments that are now in use or likely to be used in future.

The Guide is meant for the "practitioners," i.e. committed medical teachers who are running the assessment system in their respective medical schools. In addition, we believe the Curriculum and Assessment Committee members will also find this a useful source of information.

The most difficult part in developing the Guide was deciding how much detail to include. Explaining in greater detail, while desirable, risks sacrificing user friendliness. After careful deliberation we have resorted to brevity. However, we have referenced each section with pertinent articles and Internet links to allow readers access to further information. Many of these articles are *freely available* and we strongly encourage readers to review them.

Section 1 of the Guide provides a broad overview of the basic concepts and terminologies used in student assessment. Sections 2, 3, and 4 describe the advantages, limitations, psychometric properties, and examples of various assessment instruments. We also suggest recommended uses and practices based on feasibility and practicality. In formulating these recommendations, we have taken into account the general level of training of faculty members in most medical schools.

We believe assessment is a process that should *not* be taken in isolation. As we promote holistic healthcare, we should remember that the assessment system is tightly linked to other components of the curriculum, namely learning outcomes and instructional methods. We should harmonize and implement our assessment system together with these other components.

Finally, a request to all readers: despite our careful attention there might be inadvertent omissions and errors. Please point these out to us for correction and future inclusion.

Zubair Amin, Chong Yap Seng, Khoo Hoon Eng
Medical Education Unit
Yong Loo Lin School of Medicine
National University of Singapore

Disclaimer

Assessment of medical students is a technical and sophisticated process. This guide is meant to be only a practical *guide*, not an exhaustive reference source. We have only reviewed and presented selected assessment instruments. There are other assessment instruments that can be used in student assessment.

No assessment instrument is perfect. Many factors determine the success of an assessment instrument, including faculty training, curriculum planning, and quality assurance processes. Readers are responsible for the results obtained in applying the assessment methods described herein.

Contents

SECTION 1

Principles and Purpose of Assessment

CHAPTER 1

Assessment in Medical Education: An Overview

"Assessment Drives Learning"

This classic statement by George E. Miller (1919–1998) encapsulates in a single phrase the central role of assessment in any form of education. Particularly in medical education where the stakes are high, it is impossible to overstate the importance of assessment. Yet, medical schools are some of the most conservative in their choice of assessment methods, eschewing the new and embracing the tried and "tested" instead.

Traditionally, assessment is viewed as a "necessary evil" in the curriculum — an act that we carry out because we have to. We posit that assessment, properly planned and implemented, has a powerful *positive steering effect* on learning and the curriculum. It conveys what we value as important and acts as the most cogent motivator of student learning.

Assessment also fills the gaps in instruction and the curriculum. This is particularly true in large institutions and in the complex system of clinical training. In these settings, students rotate through various hospitals and departments and encounter many teachers. A robust assessment system brings an enforced level of uniformity to the curriculum.

All faculty involved in assessing and teaching students must be aware of the profound influence they have on the education of their charges. It is not the marks they give the students that matter but their choice of assessment methods, implementation, monitoring, and, above all, the effort they put into the process that truly determine the outcome of our educational system.

It is the duty of academics involved in assessments to be fully cognizant of the instruments available to them as well as the strengths and shortcomings of each. This Practical Guide seeks to give the faculty a better understanding of the principles of assessment, as well as an overview of the assessment methods available.

Purpose Driven Assessment

Assessment, if conducted properly, serves multiple purposes. Some of the purposes of medical student assessment are:

- To determine whether the learning objectives that are set *a priori* are met
- Support of student learning
- Certification and judgment of competency
- Development and evaluation of teaching programs
- Understanding of the learning process
- Predicting future performance

(Amin & Khoo, 2004; Newble, 1998)

Multiple purposes lead to wide ranging implications. One of these implications is that many stakeholders become interested in the results or data generated from the assessment. The areas of interest among the stakeholders also vary.

Stakeholders and their questions regarding assessment

Stakeholders	Questions	Interest
Medical student	• Have I achieved knowledge and competence? • How can I do better?	• Competency judgment • Support of learning
Medical teacher	• How successful was my teaching? • How can I do better?	• Program validation • Program improvement
Professional body and public (consumer)	• Are we producing safe doctors?	• Certification and licensing
Medical school	• Is the money worth spending? • Are we teaching the right things? • Are we teaching in the right way?	• Program justification • Curricular modifications • Curricular improvement

What is at Stake?

In designing and planning assessments, it is critical to keep in mind the stakes of the assessment. The purpose of the assessment will determine the stakes. Generally, formative assessments tend to be low stake, continuous assessments of low or medium stake, and summative assessments of medium to high stake.

The higher the stake is, the greater will be the consequences of the outcome of the assessment. Thus, there is a stronger need to ensure that the assessment is fair, reliable, valid, and properly conducted.

Assessment types and their characteristics

	Low Stake	Medium Stake	High Stake
Examples	Formative assessment	Continuous assessment (CA), end of posting test; house officer evaluation	Professional examination
Decisions and consequences	Few, easily reversible decisions, low consequence	Decisions can be reversed	Decisions are generally irreversible, consequences high
Developmental effort needed	Low	Medium	High
Quality assurance	Seldom needed	Recommended	Required
Monitoring and implementation	Individual level	Departmental level	Central; faculty or medical school level
Check for validity and reliability	Not routinely required	Recommended	Required

Examples of useful assessment instruments in low stakes examination include long essay questions and "traditional" long case examination. However, their use in high stakes examination is undesirable, as they tend to lack a high degree of reliability and are inherently prone to marking errors. A better strategy for high stakes examinations would be to replace those with more objective assessment instruments such as multiple short answer questions (in place of long essay questions) and objective structured clinical examination (in place of the traditional long case).

Low Stake Examinations		High Stake Examinations
Long essay question	⟶	Multiple short answer question
Traditional long case	⟶	Multi-station OSCE

References and Further Reading

"Assessment drives learning"

McGUIRE, C. (1999) George E Miller, MD, 1919–1998, *Med. Edu.* 33: 312–314.

Purpose driven assessment

AMIN, Z. & KHOO, H.E. (2003) Overview of Assessment and Evaluation. In: *Basics in Medical Education*, 251–260 (World Scientific Publishing Company, Singapore).

NEWBLE, D. (1998) Assessment. In: Jolly, B. & Rees, L. (eds.) *Medical Education in the Millennium*, 131–142 (Oxford University Press, Oxford, UK).

What is at stake?

SHEPARD, E. & GODWIN, J. (2004) Assessments through the learning process, Question *mark* White Paper. Questionmark Corporation. Web address: http://questionmark.com/us/home.htm; (last accessed December 2005).

CHAPTER 2

Key Concepts in Assessment

Formative and Summative Assessment

Formative assessment is *process focused*; its primary purpose is to provide feedback to both student and teacher while the program is still ongoing. Formative assessment tends to be low stakes examinations. Formative assessment is an important component in education as good formative assessment with feedback improves student learning and leads to better performance in summative assessment.

Summative assessment is *outcome focused*; its primary purpose is to determine the achievement of the student or the program. Summative assessments are generally high stakes examinations and require substantial developmental effort and strict quality control.

Validity

Validity is one of the key psychometric properties of an assessment instrument. It determines whether an assessment instrument really tests what it is supposed to test.

The concept of validity may be further expanded into the following:

Content validity: *Representativeness* of learning objectives in the assessment. In practice this is achieved by blueprinting (see below). For example, a surgical trainee should be tested on his/her surgical skills and not just knowledge of pathology.

Construct validity: Congruence of assessment instrument with the purpose. For example, communication skills should be tested by direct observation of the interview between the candidate and the patient and not by a paper and pencil test.

Predictive validity: Ability of the instrument to predict future performance. For example, the relationship between the performance in the final M.B.B.S examination and performance during training as a house officer.

Face validity: Acceptability of the instrument to the users (students, teachers) in determining its usefulness to measure what it is supposed to measure.

For practical purposes, validity is determined by either a judgmental approach by experts (e.g. content validity) or by an empirical data driven approach (e.g. predictive validity).

Blueprinting

Blueprinting refers to the process where test content is carefully planned against the learning objectives. The examination blueprint specifies the objectives that are to be tested in the given examination as well as their relative weight on the examination. A proper blueprint is the first crucial step in developing a valid examination and must not be overlooked. A proper blueprint will ensure fair representation of all the important curricular objectives in the examination.

The scope and structure of the blueprint will depend on the nature of the examination. For example, for a final examination, in a centrally administered integrated curriculum the test blueprint would take into account all the core learning objectives and physician tasks.

Below is a simplified step-by-step approach to developing a test blueprint in an integrated curriculum:

1. Create a table with major systems (cardiovascular, respiratory, etc.) on the top row and physician tasks (history taking, data interpretation, management, etc.) on the left-most column
2. Determine the major disease or presenting problem of interest for each system
3. Determine the weight to be assigned to each problem
4. Map the physician's task against the disease or presenting problem
5. Make sure that there is a cross-mark for each column and each row

System → Physician Task ↓	CVS	Respiratory	GIT	Renal	CNS
History taking	X		X		
Physical examination		X			X
Data interpretation				X	
Disease management			X	X	
Prevention	X				
Pathophysiology		X			
Epidemiology	X				

	CVS	Respiratory	GIT	Renal	CNS
History taking	Chest Pain		Rectal bleeding		
Physical examination		Breathlessness			Hemi-paresis
Data interpretation				Acute oliguria	
Disease management			Epigastric pain (PUD)	Dysuria (UTI)	
Prevention	Hyper-cholesterolemia				
Pathophysiology		Asthma			
Epidemiology	Hypertension				

	CVS	Respiratory	GIT	Renal	CNS
History taking	OSCE		OSCE		
Physical examination		OSCE			OSCE
Data interpretation				Written test	
Disease management			Written test	Written test	
Prevention	Written test				
Pathophysiology		OSCE			
Epidemiology	Written test				

Fig. 1 A simplified approach to examination blueprint development in an integrated curriculum.

6. Determine the most suitable method for testing the task (e.g. MCQ or OSCE)
7. Assign faculty member to develop test questions for each task

Often the core content of the curriculum is used for course blueprinting. The Medical Council of Canada makes available the objectives of its qualifying examination in its website http://www.mcc.ca/Objectives_online/. This can be referred to during the development of the blueprint.

Suggestions for Improving Validity

- Use content blueprint to assign and design the questions
- Focus on the important; i.e., core components in the curriculum
- Sample widely
  - Across content
  - Across domains of interest (e.g., knowledge, skills, and behavior)
- Choose an instrument that most resembles the task that a physician is required to perform
- Choose multiple instruments to have a valid assessment

Reliability

Reliability usually refers to consistency of a test over time, over different cases (inter-case), and different examiners (inter-rater).

Inter-rater reliability: It measures the consistency of rating of performance by different examiners (raters) keeping all the other variables as consistent as possible.

Inter-case reliability: It measures a candidate's performance from one case to another keeping all the other variables as consistent as possible.

Test-retest reliability: An indicator of consistency over time.

Reliability can be determined statistically using several methods. Test-retest reliability is measured by the correlation of one score with the others. The score ranges from 0 (low reliability) to 1 (high reliability). Inter-rater reliability compares scores between different examiners. Internal consistency (intra-exam, inter-item) is measured by Cronbach alpha. The range of value can be 0 (low consistency) to 1 (high consistency).

Some reliability guidelines
0.90 = high reliability
0.80 = medium reliability
0.70 = low reliability

In general, the reliability of an examination improves with increasing testing time and number of questions. In other words, for a particular format, a three-hour-long examination would result in better reliability than a one-hour-long examination using the same format. For example, in one study, the reliability of a one-hour-long MCQ-based paper was 0.62. This improved to 0.76 for a 2-hour-long examination and reached 0.93 for a 3-hour-long examination (Norcini *et al.*, 1985).

Suggestions for Improving Validity

- Do not depend on shorter tests
  - A 15-station OSCE will result in a more reliable test than a 5-station OSCE
- Consider efficiency in time, grading effort, and test format
  - For the same testing time, MCQ will give more reliable results than essay questions
- Design the test to sample broadly across the domains of interest
- Vary the difficulty level of questions
  - To help differentiate between good and poorly performing students
  - To help determine the pass/fail boundary

Relationship between Validity and Reliability

Reliability and validity are closely linked. Reliability is a necessary prerequisite of a valid test. Validity is severely compromised in an unreliable test. Conversely, a test can be highly reliable (consistent) without being valid.

Feasibility (Cost and Acceptability)

Ideal assessments may not always be possible because of constraints in resources. Some of the constraints in resources that are very pertinent to medical education and need to be considered in detail are:

- Availability of examiners
- Time to develop the test
- Time to administer the test
- Time to grade and analyze the papers
- Costs associated with administration of the site, and
- Faculty training

Utility of an Assessment Instrument

The utility, or the practical usefulness of an assessment instrument, depends on its relative advantages, uses, and limits. It has to be a considered judgment on the part of examiners to decide which assessment instrument is best suited for the purpose.

Thus, the utility of an assessment instrument is based on careful consideration of several factors: reliability, validity, educational impact, costs, and acceptability of the method (Shuwirth & van der Vleuten, 2004).

For example, in an admission exercise to medical school, the overriding concern from the perspective of the administrators is to have a highly reliable tool; the educational impact of the tool is of less concern. Similarly, instruments that we use for on-the-job performance assessment need to have a very high educational value in supporting students' learning; reliability in such situations may not be the primary consideration.

References and Further Reading

Reliability

NORCINI, J.J., SWANSON, D.B., GROSSO, L.J. & WEBSTER, G.D. (1985) Reliability, validity and efficiency of multiple choice question and patient management problem item formats in assessment of clinical competence, *Med. Edu.* 19(3): 238–247.

RUDNER, L.M-S. & WILLIAM, D. (2001) Reliability. In: *ERIC Digest.* ERIC Identifier: ED458213; Web address: http://www.ericdigests.org/2002-2/reliability.htm (last accessed December 2005).

Utility of an assessment instrument

SCHUWIRTH, L.W.T. & VLEUTEN van der, C. (2004) Changing education, changing assessment, changing research? *Med. Edu.* 38(8): 805–812.

CHAPTER 3

Special Issues in Assessment in Clinical Medicine

Context Specificity

The evidence from cognitive psychology and research in clinical competence and expertise suggests that there is *no* generic problem solving and cognitive skill (Norman, 2003). The corollary to this proposition is that performance in a specific problem area (e.g., a patient management problem) does not tell much about the performance of the candidate in other problem areas. To further extend the theme, a candidate's performance during the examination with an asthma patient may have a poor correlation with the same candidate's performance in other situations, for example, the management of rheumatoid arthritis.

This is a very significant finding with overarching ramifications in test design. We cannot judge, with confidence, the competency of a candidate based on his/her performance in only one clinical encounter. The only practical way of eliminating context specificity is to employ multiple sampling strategies, including multiple cases, multiple raters, and multiple items to achieve a broader perspective of the candidate's performance.

Generalizability of Assessment Data

Somewhat related to the theme of context specificity is *generalizability*. This refers to applicability of the results of an assessment to more than the sample of cases or test questions that was used in a specific assessment. In other words, generalizability tells us how confident we are in predicting the performance of the candidate beyond the encounters that take place in the examination. By applying the generalizability theory, it is also possible to examine how different aspects of observation — such as using different raters, using different types of instruments, or testing under different conditions — can affect the dependability of the scores (Pellegrino, Chudowsky, & Glasser, 2001).

The generalizability co-efficient is a statistical estimate of *reproducibility* of measurement. It varies from 0.1 to 1.0 (Wass *et al.*, 2001).

A co-efficient of 0.8 is seen as the minimum requirement for reliable measurement.

Context Specificity and the Problem of Generalizability

Clinical competence in medicine is a complex phenomenon. Multiple skills interplay with each other to result in a composite expression of what we know as clinical competence. Some of these skills are history taking, problem solving, diagnostic reasoning, decision-making, and communication.

A consistent finding in the literature is that there is *no* generic skill involved in clinical competence. In other words, there is no generic problem solving, clinical decision making, or patient management skill that is transferable across all the domains of competence (Epstein & Hundert, 2002; Norman, 2003). Performance in one domain of clinical competence has very little correlation with performance in other domains.

Similarly, performance in one case or with one patient has poor reproducibility to similar performances in another case or patient with dissimilar problems. Dr Arthur Elstein (1978) coined the term *case specificity* to describe this observation and since then it has been confirmed many times (Norcini, 2002). In simpler terms, a candidate's ability to deal competently with a patient with rheumatoid arthritis does not mean he or she is equally competent in dealing with a patient with diabetes mellitus.

This phenomenon of poor correlation across cases is evident regardless of the method of assessment used (Norman, 2003). It is equally evident with *single* objective structured clinical examinations (OSCE) station, *single* long or short case, or *single* oral examination. In other words, an OSCE with a single station is no better than a structured long case with a single patient. Both are equally faulty with poor and inadequate sampling.

A very important consequence of this finding is that we need to sample candidates across *multiple* domains of clinical skills, and with *multiple* problems or patients, in order to have a valid and reliable test with generalizable results.

Why do we need multiple sampling in assessment?

Multiple sampling across different skills and domains of interest, with different patients and clinical scenarios, and with different examiners is essential to have a valid and reliable examination. There are several very convincing arguments and empirical evidence to support this.

- Clinical competency in medicine is *highly context and problem specific*. There is no generic problem solving skill. The problem solving skill in one specific situation does not translate into equal competency in another situation. Competency in one particular situation cannot be generalized to other situations. To address the issue of context specificity, we need to design tests that allow multiple sampling so that we can be reasonably confident about the candidate's competency in a range of clinical situations.
- Systematic error from single encounter based examinations (e.g., single long case with or without viva, single essay question) has been extensively researched and documented. The reliability of such a test is generally poor. Much of the variation in marking is often the result of "extraneous noise" rather than "true signal." It is estimated that the reliability of single long case with viva can be as low as 0.39, meaning that almost two-thirds of the variation in the marking is the result of factors not associated with competency of the candidate in that given situation.
- Multiple sampling strategies (e.g. multiple clinical situations with multiple examiners) also minimize the inter-examiner or inter-rater variability. Inter-rater variability exists even in the best assessment situation.

(*Continued*)

(*Continued*)

Interventions such as faculty training and standardization of the marking scheme do not eliminate the inter-rater biases. Multiple sampling with multiple well-informed examiners, if applied along with standardised marking schemes and other good practices in assessment, will minimize the bias significantly.

Most of the accepted methods used in assessment in clinical competency now utilize multiple sampling strategies. Examples of assessment methods that use such strategies include multi-station Objective Structured Clinical Examination (over single long case), and multiple short answer questions (over one or a few long essay questions). Many newer performance assessment methods such as mini-CEX, Directly Observed Procedural Skills (DOPS), Clinical Work Sampling (CWS), and 360-degree evaluation also employ multiple sampling strategies.

References and Further Reading

Context specificity

NORMAN, G. (2003) Postgraduate assessment — reliability and validity, *Trans.: J. Coll. Med. S. Afri.* 47: 71–75.

Generalizability of assessment data

MEDICAL COUNCIL OF CANADA. (2004) Objectives of qualifying examination, 3rd ed. Web address: http://www.mcc.ca/Objectives_online/ (last accessed December 2005).

PELLEGRINO, J.W., CHUDOWSKY, N., & GLASSER, R. (2001) (Eds.) Contribution of measurement and statistical modelling of assessment. In: *Knowing What Students Know the Science and Design of Educational Assessment* (National Academy Press, Washington, DC, USA).

WOJTCZAK, A. (2002) Glossary of medical education terms. Institute of International Medical Education. Web address: http://www.iime.org/glossary.htm#C (last accessed December 2005).

Context specificity and the problem of generalizability

ELSTEIN, A.S., SHULMAN, L.S., & SPRAFKA, S.A. (1978) *Medical Problem-solving: An Analysis of Clinical Reasoning* (Cambridge, MA, USA, Harvard University Press).

EPSTEIN, R.M. & HUNDERT, E.M. (2002) Defining and assessing clinical competence, *JAMA* 387: 226–235.

NORCINI, J.J. (2002) The death of the long case?, *BMJ* **324**: 408–409.

NORMAN, G. (2003) Postgraduate assessment — reliability and validity, *Trans: J. Coll. Med. S. Afri.* 47(4): 71–75.

CHAPTER 4
Standard Setting

A standard is a special score that serves as the boundary between those who perform well and those who do not. It is a systematic way of gathering value judgments, reaching consensus, and expressing that consensus as a single score on a test. As this involves judgment, the credibility of the standard would vary according to who sets the standards, the characteristics of the methods used, and the outcome (Norcini, 2003).

Norm Referenced Standard

This is based on the assumption that the test scores are distributed normally and the scores of a given student are compared with the scores of other students. Norm-referenced standard takes into account other students' performance in deciding on the pass or fail grade for a given student. Therefore, in a hypothetical situation where the majority of the students are poor performers, it is possible for a given student to be deemed to have passed even when his/her performance falls short of the desired competency; i.e. in this situation it gives a "false-positive test" result. Conversely, if the group's performance is high, then there is a high likelihood that a given candidate might be unfairly judged to fail in the examination, even when his/her performance has reached the desired level. In this situation, a "false-negative result" is likely.

Recommended use: Admission exercise which requires selection of a predetermined number of candidates.

Criterion Referenced Standard

This is based on predefined test goals and standards in performance during an examination where a certain level of knowledge or skill has been determined as required for passing. In performance-based examinations, criterion reference standard is the preferred mode of making pass/fail cut-off points. The pass-fail decision about a particular candidate's performance is made independently of other candidates' performance.

Standard setting in the criterion-referenced method often requires more technical expertise. There are many published methods of reaching a desired standard, including the test-centered approach (e.g. Angoff's method and its variations); examinee-centered approach (e.g. borderline group method); and several other innovations. It is not within the scope of this Guide to present a detailed technical discussion of the standard setting; readers are requested to consult the references below.

Recommended use: Competency- or performance-based examination.

References and Further Reading

FRIEDMAN BEN-DAVID, M. (2000) Standard setting in student assessment, Education Guide 18 (Association for Medical Education in Europe, AMEE, Scotland, UK).

NORCINI, J.J. (2003) Setting standard on educational test, *Med. Edu.* 37: 464–469.

WASS, V., VLEUTEN, van der C., SHATZER, J., & JONES, R. (2001) Assessment of clinical competence, *The Lancet* 357: 945–949.

CHAPTER 5

A Model for Assessment

George Miller (1990) proposed a schema, "Miller's Pyramid," which proposes clinical competence in multiple levels: "Knows," "Knows How," "Shows," and "Does." A candidate "knows" first before progressing to "knows how." In other words, "knows" is analogous to factual knowledge and "knows how" is equivalent to concept building and understanding. At a higher level, a candidate "shows how" i.e. develops the competence to "perform." At the highest level, the candidate "does" i.e. actually carries out the concerned tasks competently in real life situations.

It is convenient to use this schema while choosing an assessment instrument for an examination, although one must acknowledge that separation of clinical competence from one level to another is artificial, and knowledge and clinical competence is a holistic entity.

Assessment instruments *vary considerably* in their uses to test different levels of competence. For example, while multiple choice questions (MCQ) are highly efficient for testing "knows" or "knowledge," its use in assessing "shows how" or "does" is limited. Similarly, OSCEs, although efficient in assessing "shows how," are rather impractical if one wants to test a large amount of knowledge at the lower "knows" level.

As such, it is imperative that when planning an assessment system for clinical competence, we choose at least one or two assessment instruments from each of these levels to develop a composite representation of the candidate's ability.

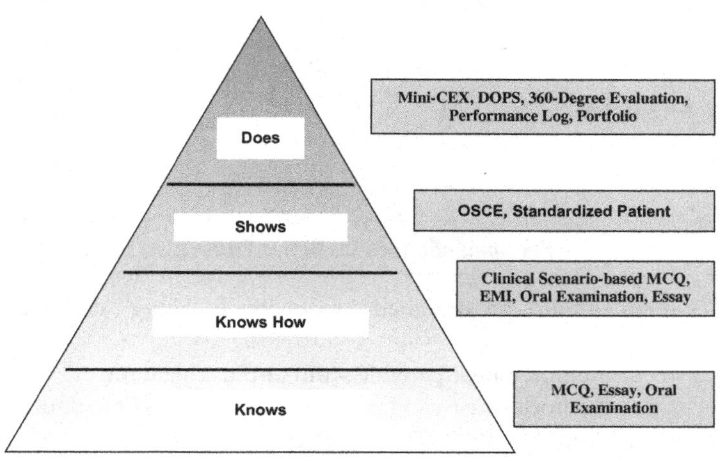

Assessment level	Examples
Knows and Knows How	• Oral Examination • Long Essay Question • Short Essay Question • Multiple Choice Questions • Extended Matching Items (EMI) • Key Features Examination
Shows How	• OSCE • Long Case • Short Case
Does	• Mini Clinical Evaluation Exercise (mini-CEX) • Direct Observation of Procedural Skills (DOPS) • Checklist • 360-Degree Evaluation • Logbook • Portfolio

> *No single assessment method can provide all the data required for judgment of anything so complex as the delivery of professional services by a successful physician.*
>
> George Miller 1990

Recommendations for Better Practice

- Assessment should be designed prospectively along with learning outcomes
- Assessment methods must provide valid and usable data
- Assessment methods must yield reliable and generalizable data
- Assessment should be driven by the purpose in mind
- Multiple assessment instruments targeting all levels in Miller's pyramid are necessary to capture a reasonable breadth of competency
- Content validity is best achieved by a proper blueprint of learning outcomes
- Students need to be tested with multiple cases and scenarios to achieve an acceptable degree of reliability
- For summative assessment, the standard of the examination should be based on criterion-based referencing

References and Further Reading

LYNCH, D.C. & SWING, S.T. Key considerations for selecting assessment instruments and implementing assessment systems, Accreditation Council of Graduate Medical Education (ACGME). Web address: http://www.acgme.org/outcome/assess/keyConsider.asp (last accessed December 2005).

MILLER, G.E. (1990) The assessment of clinical skills/competence/performance, *Acad. Med.* 65(9): S63–S67.

WOJTCZAK, A. (2002) Glossary of medical education terms, Institute of International Medical Education (IIME), Web address: http://www.iime.org/glossary.htm (last accessed December 2005).

SECTION 2

Assessment of "Knows" and "Knows How"

CHAPTER 6

Oral Examination/Viva

Description

In an oral examination, a candidate faces one or more examiners who ask questions. Examiners might use a blueprint to select content area and a structured marking scheme. Often, oral examinations are conducted in conjunction with long or short cases.

Limitations of Traditional Viva

- Poor content validity
- High inter-rater variability
- Inconsistency in marking
- Lack of standardization of questions
- Tends to test factual knowledge rather than higher order knowledge such as problem solving

Use With Borderline Candidates

- As the instrument is prone to biases and is inherently unreliable, it is not recommended for use during high stakes situations such as judging a borderline candidate (Wass *et al.*, 2001).

Cited Advantage

- The ability to recall and synthesise information can be done through face-to-face interactions.

Pertinent Evidence

- It would take 12–16 case histories in oral examinations to achieve the acceptable degree of 0.8 generalizability according to Swanson's study (as cited in Wass *et al.*, 2001)
- Reported reliability of oral examinations in 4 hours of testing time is only 0.5 (Wass *et al.*, 2001)
- The presence of more examiners asking limited questions produces better reliability as compared to a single examiner asking multiple questions, according to Swanson's study (1987)
- Examiners are more likely to disagree in the case of borderline candidates with regards to pass/fail decisions (Waugh & Moyse, 1969)
- Inter-rater agreement in scoring during one session does not necessarily mean reliability (Campbell & Murray, 1995) as agreement in the scores of a candidate's performance across different sessions can be still low

Possible Uses

- Exploration of complex ethical issues (Wass *et al.*, 2001)
- Assessment of attitudinal issues (Wass *et al.*, 2001)
- As part of formative assessment exercises

Practical Tips

Several practical measures may improve slightly the validity and reliability of viva examinations (although it might be impractical and even impossible to reach an acceptable degree of reliability and validity) in situations where oral examinations need to be continued as a summative assessment (Davis & Karunathilake, 2005):

(a) Structure the oral examination
(b) Use content blueprint
(c) Standardize questions and answers
(d) Use independent and multiple raters
(e) Use multiple sessions

Recommended practice	Effect and rationale
Oral examinations should not be used in high stakes examination	Unreliable and invalid
Oral examinations should not be used in making pass/fail decisions with borderline candidates	Instruments with higher reliability should be used instead

References and Further Reading

CAMPBELL, L.M. & MURRAY, T.S. (1995) Improving oral examination, *BMJ* **311**: 1572–1573.

KARUNATHILAKE, I. & DAVIS, M. (2005) The place of oral examination in today's assessment system, *Med. Teacher* **27**(4): 294–297.

SWANSON, D. (1987). A measurement framework for performance based test. In: HART, I.R. & HARDEN, R.M. (eds.), *Further Developments in Assessing Clinical Competence*, 13–15 (Montreal Can–Heal), Cited in Val Wass, 2001.

WASS, V., VLEUTEN, van der C., SHATZER, J. & JONES, R. (2001) Assessment of clinical competence, *The Lancet* **357**: 945–949.

WAUGH, D. & MOYSE, C.A. (1969) Oral examination: A videotape study of the reproducibility of grades in pathology, *Can. Med. Assoc. J.* **100**: 635–640.

CHAPTER 7

Long Essay Questions (LEQ)

Description

Typically a long essay is a piece of prose that varies in length from several paragraphs to several pages. The question stem often contains a phrase such as: "Describe the management of ...".

Scoring of the essay questions deserves special attention especially in the context of an examination. Two methods of scoring are generally employed: analytic (point-scoring) method or global scoring method. The analytic method is more useful in focused essay question (see example below). In the analytic method, the model answer is broken down into several portions and marks are assigned to each content area. A predetermined structured marking scheme and use of multiple raters further improves the reliability.

In global scoring, the examiner reads the entire essay and makes a global (holistic) judgment about the quality. Global scoring may be in the form of a letter (e.g. A to E) or Likert scale-type (e.g. fail, borderline fail, fair, good, excellent). Cashin (1987) suggested a method of global scoring. According to his suggestion, examiners read all the essays quickly and sort them into piles of different grades. Then the examiner re-reads each pile to ensure that each essay has been accurately (fairly) assigned to that pile.

Strengths of Essay Questions

- Assessment of complex learning situations that cannot be assessed by other means
- Assessment of writing skills and the ability to present arguments succinctly and coherently

- Unlike the MCQ or other forms of objective test, essay questions cannot be answered by looking at the choices

Limitations

- Poor representation of content; unable to test broad domains of knowledge
- Pursuing objectivity by "over-structuring" the question may trivialize the question and therefore compromise objectivity (Schuwirth & van der Vleuten, 2003)
- Poor reliability and inconsistency in marking
- Time consuming and difficult to mark; inefficient

In general, a large number of essay questions are required to have a good breadth in content coverage, making it very impractical in terms of time spent in administering and grading the examination.

Recommended Use

- Assessment at level of "knows how" with complex situations such as discussion of medico-legal and ethical issues

Evidence

- Research by the American Board of Internal Medicine (ABIM) shows that essay questions capture only a small aspect of medical competence over and above that measured by MCQ (Day *et al.*, 1990)
- In the same study, with analytic scoring only 6% of variance in test score was related to essay questions. With global scoring the corresponding number is only 5%, indicating that essay questions provide little extra information about the variability of a candidate's performance (Day *et al.*, 1990)
- Research by the ABIM with stringent marking criteria and standardization shows that using analytical scoring systems, the generalizability coefficient of an essay test with 12 questions (requiring 3 hours of testing time) is 0.36. It was estimated that to reach

an acceptable generalizability coefficient of 0.80 it would require 72 essay items or almost 18 hours of testing time (Norcini, 1990)
- With global scoring, although the generalizability coefficient is improved, it would still require 22 essay questions or 5.5 hours of essay time to reach an acceptable coefficient of 0.80 (Norcini *et al.*, 1990)

Examples

Non-focused essay; undesirable

Discuss informed consent and its medico-legal implication in the context of health care.

Focused essay question; desirable

(a) Describe the role and responsibility of a doctor taking informed consent
(b) Give examples (up to three) of situations where informed consent is not routinely required
(c) Provide examples (up to three) of situations where informed consent could be deemed invalid

Recommended practice	Effect and rationale
Long essay questions (LEQ) should not be used in high stakes examination	Unreliable, poor content validity
Use multiple short essay questions instead	Better content validity
Use clinical scenario-based modified essay questions	Tests higher level of knowledge
Design essay questions that focus on a few specific, important learning objectives	More focused, better reliability, easier to mark
Use of structured predefined marking scheme	Improves reliability of marking

References and Further Reading

CASHIN, W.E. (1987) Improving essay tests. Idea Paper No. 17, Center for Faculty Evaluation and Development. Kansas State University, Kansas, USA. Web address: http://www.idea.ksu.edu/papers/Idea_Paper_17.pdf (last accessed December 2005).

DAY, S.C., NORCINI, J.J., DISERENS, D. *et al.* (1990) The validity of an essay test of clinical judgment, *Acad. Med.* **65**(9): S39–S40.

NORCINI, J.J., DISERENS, D., DAY, S.C. *et al.* (1990) The scoring and reproducibility of an essay test of clinical judgment, *Acad. Med.* **65**(9): S41–S42.

SCHUWIRTH, L.W.T. & VLEUTEN, C.P.M. (2003) Written assessment. In: Cantillon P, Hutchison L, and Wood D (eds.) *ABC of Learning and Teaching in Medicine*, 29–31 (BMJ Publishing Group, UK).

CHAPTER 8

Short Answer Questions (SAQ)

Description

A practical alternative to the long essay question, the short answer question is an open ended, semi-structured question format. A structured, pre-determined marking scheme improves objectivity. The questions can incorporate clinical scenarios.

A similar format is also known as modified essay question (MEQ) or constructed response question (CRQ).

Advantages

- Better content coverage as compared to long essay question
- Improved objectivity as the marking scheme can be structured and predetermined
- Less laborious to mark
- Higher chance for assessment of clinical reasoning

Limitation

- If a large amount of knowledge needs to be tested, it is more efficient to use MCQs

Evidence

- Equal or higher test reliabilities can be achieved with fewer SAQs as compared to true/false items (ten Cate, 1996, 1997 cited by Rademakers, ten Cate, & Bär, 2005)

Suggested Uses

- Medium stakes progress test
- End of posting knowledge test

Example

The following structure of SAQ is based on the University Medical Centre, Utrecht School of Medical Science, the Netherlands (developed by ten Cate and J Rademakers)

Case vignette

You are a medical officer in pediatrics. You are asked to review a one-hour-old baby for increasing respiratory rate and sub-costal retraction. The baby was born at 35 weeks to a 29-year-old mother via elective LSCS. The indication for LSCS was uncontrolled BP. The mother had regular follow-up during her antenatal period. She had gestational diabetes and pre-eclamsia.

Question 1: What are the most likely diagnoses? (Name two)
Question 2: What are the preliminary investigations that you would like to perform at this point? (Name three)
Question 3: For each of the diagnoses list one primary pathophysiological mechanism.

Model answer:

Question 1: Hyaline membrane disease; transient tachypnea of newborn (TTNB); (two marks)
Question 2: Full blood count; chest X-ray; and arterial blood gas (three marks)
Question 3: deficiency of surfactant; failure to reabsorb lung fluid (two marks)

Practical Tips in Writing SAQ

- Choose a case vignette related to the physician's tasks
- Link the questions directly to the case vignette
- Ensure that questions cannot be answered without the case

- Specify the number of responses
- Specify the mark assigned to each question
- Incorporate basic science principles (e.g. pathophysiology, mechanism of action) in the clinical vignette

Recommended practice	Effect and rationale
Use SAQ as an alternative to long essay questions	Better content validity and reliability
Use content blueprint	Better representation of content; decreases the chance of overlap with other questions format
If a large body of knowledge needs to be tested use MCQ instead	MCQ is more efficient in testing large body of knowledge
Use of structured predetermined marking scheme	Improves reliability of marking
Link questions to the case scenario	Better representation of clinical competency

References and Further Reading

RADEMAKERS, J., ten CATE, TH. J., & BÄR, P.R. (2005) Progress testing with short answer questions, *Med. Teacher* 27(7): 578–582.

CHAPTER 9

Multiple Choice Questions (MCQ)

Description

The MCQ is a restricted response, objective assessment instrument. It contains:

- a stem or a description of a problem
- lead-in or the question, and
- options list

Advantages

- Assessment of a large amount of knowledge in a relatively short time
- Contextualization with clinical vignette and scenario (see example below) to improve validity
- Can be made reliable and objective
- Computerized marking is possible

Limitations

- Good quality MCQs are relatively difficult to construct
- Prone to cuing and technical error

Best Evidence and Practice

- Reported reliability of a 4-hour long MCQ paper is >0.90, thus exceeding the requirements for a reliable test (Val Wass *et al.*, 2001)

- Reported reproducibility of a 90-item MCQ paper is 0.88 (Norcini, 2002)
- Faculty training improves quality of MCQs (Jozefiwicz *et al.*, 2002)
- Good true/false items are difficult to develop and tend to test lower order factual knowledge (Case & Swanson, 2002)

Examples

Non-contextual MCQ (isolated fact version; should be avoided in examination)
In erythropoietin deficiency, you are expected to see the following pattern in RBC morphology:

(a) Normocytic normochromic
(b) Microcytic normochromic
(c) Macrocytic normochromic
(d) Microcytic hypochromic
(e) None of the above

Non-contextual MCQ (isolated fact version; should be avoided in examination)
Which of the following hematopoietic factors is produced by the kidney?

(a) Rennin
(b) Angiotensin
(c) Erythropoietin
(d) Aldosterone
(e) Cortisol

Note that both examples test knowledge that is important but in an isolated manner. Students only need to have recall-type knowledge to answer correctly.

Contextual MCQ with the same themes (better example)

A 55-year-old patient with chronic renal failure undergoing dialysis. He appears to be pale. A full blood count shows the following red cell indices:

Hemoglobin: 8.7 gm/dl
Hematocrit: 26%
MCV: 92 fL (expected range 80-100 fL)
MCH: 33 pg (expected range 27-31 pg)
MCHC: 33 gm/dl (expected range 32-36 gm/dl)
Reticulocyte count: 0.2%

Which of the following is the most appropriate therapy?

(a) Erythropoietin
(b) Ferrous sulphate
(c) Folic acid
(d) Vitamin B 6
(e) Vitamin B 12 (cyanocobalamin)

Note the following features in this MCQ

- Combines basic science knowledge with clinical science knowledge
- Students need to connect multiple themes (in this case the role of the kidney in erythropoiesis and the changes in RBC morphology)
- The lead-in (question) focuses on only one aspect of the condition
- The MCQ can be answered without looking at the option (cover test)

Recommended practice	Effect and rationale
Use of blueprint	Improves content validity
Context or clinical scenario-based MCQ	Assessment of higher order knowledge in "knows how" level
Use a standard checklist (see below) prior to submission of MCQ	Efficient in identifying the problem and providing feedback to the item-writer
Invite peers to review the question	Peer review will detect subtle hidden problems
Analyze MCQ by difficulty and discriminatory indices	Quality assurance
Avoid true/false item format	Reduces negative effect of learning

Imprecise and Difficult Terms to Avoid in MCQ

Several terms, sadly not infrequently used in MCQ, should be avoided while writing MCQ as they are imprecise, difficult to quantify, and give away clue to the correct answer. Examples of such words are:

- Never
- Always
- Sometime
- Generally
- Commonly
- Usually
- Same as
- Can be
- May be
- Can appear
- Possible (possibly)

Pre-Submission Checklist for MCQ

MCQ Number:

Content Area:

Submitted by:

Overall	Yes	No	Comments
The topic is important for the learners			
The level of difficulty is appropriate			
Stem			
Stem is clear and complete			
Contains no jargon or abbreviations			
Context-based/contains integrated clinical vignette			
Tests beyond knowledge recall and memorization			
Lead-in			
Focuses on one aspect (e.g. indication, side-effects, contraindication, mechanism of action)			
Can be answered without looking at the options			
Options			
All options are uniform (length, grammatical construct)			
Options do not give clue to the answer			
No usage of ambiguous terms (e.g. almost, never, frequent)			
There is no "all of the above" or "none of the above" option			

Decision

- ☐ Accept; as it is
- ☐ Revise; minor changes (see comments below)
- ☐ Resubmit; major changes necessary (see comments below)

Comments for the item-writer

____

____

____

References and Further Reading

2006 Step 1 Content description and sample test materials (2005) Published by the Federation of State Medical Boards of the United States, Inc. and the National Board of Medical Examiners® (NBME®). Web address: http://www.usmle.org/step1/default.htm; (last accessed November 2005).

CASE, S. & SWANSON, D.B. (2002). Constructing written test for the basic and clinical sciences 3rd Ed. Published by: National Board of Medical Examiners®, Philadelphia, PA USA. Web address: http://www.nbme.org/about/itemwriting.asp (last accessed December 2005).

JOZEFOWICZ, R.F., KOEPPEN, B.M., CASE, S., GALBRAITH, R., SWANSON, D., & GLEW, R.H. (2002). The quality of in-house examination, *Acad. Med.* 77(2): 156–161.

NORCINI, J.J. (2002) The death of the long case?, *BMJ* 324(7334): 408–409. Web address: http://www.pubmedcentral.nih.gov/articlerender.fcgi?artid=65539; (last accessed December 2005).

WASS, V., VLEUTEN, ven der C., SHATZER, J., & JONES, R. (2001) Assessment of clinical competence, *The Lancet* 357: 945–949.

CHAPTER 10

Extended Matching Items (EMI)

Description

EMI is a relatively new format of objective testing which is somewhat similar to the MCQ, except that it is based on a single theme and has a long option list to avoid cuing. It is also known as extended matching question (EMQ).

Advantages

- Assessment of clinical scenarios with less cuing
- Similar objectivity and consistency as with conventional single-best item format of MCQ
- Relatively easier to construct
- Answer scripts can be made machine readable
- Question quality can be determined

Limitations

- Relatively newer format
- Need for faculty training

Evidence

- EMI is a practical alternative to MCQ while maintaining objectivity and consistency (Case & Swanson, 1993; Case & Swanson, 2002)
- EMI allows greater discrimination over limited choice MCQ as the responses are more widely distributed (Case & Swanson, 1994)

- EMI is capable of testing clinical reasoning effectively (Beullen *et al.*, 2005)

Example

Theme: Patients with sore-throat

For each of the following scenarios, choose the most likely organism

Question 1:
An 18-year-old boy presented to the general practioner with sore throat. He also complaints of fever for 4 days and malaise. On examination, his cervical lymph nodes are found to be enlarged. His girl friend has similar symptoms. His peripheral blood film shows atypical lymphocytes.

Question 2:
A 7-year-old boy presented to the pediatrician with acute onset of fever and sore throat. On examination, the tonsils are found to be swollen with creamy exudates. His cervical lymph nodes are enlarged and tender. Several of his classmates recently had similar symptoms. His full blood count shows the following WBC parameters: total white count 18,000/ml, neutrophil 84%.

a) Adenovirus
b) *Corynebacterium diphtheriae*
c) Coxsackie virus
d) Cytomegalovirus
e) Epstein-Barr virus
f) *Hemophilus influenzae*
g) Influenza virus
h) *Mycoplasma pneumoniae*
i) *Streptococcus pyogenes*
j) Rhinovirus

Suggested Answer
Question 1: e
Question 2: i

Practical Tips in Writing EMI

- Design questions that are context-based or clinical scenario-based
- Each question should be related to one single theme (e.g. diagnosis of sore throat, appropriate therapy in hypertension)
- Limit the questions for each theme to a reasonable few numbers

- Include most, if not all, possible answers (in this example, causes of sore throat) in the option list
- List the options alphabetically

Recommended practice	Effect and rationale
Use EMI in both basic science and clinical science examination	Assessment of clinical competency in "knows how"
Analyze EMI by difficulty and discriminatory indices	Important for quality assurance

References and Further Reading

BEULLEN, J., STRUVF, E., & DAMME, B.V. (2005) Do extended matching multiple choice questions measure clinical reasoning? *Med. Edu.* **39**(4): 410–415.

CASE, S.M. & SWANSON D.B. (1993) Extended matching items: A practical alternative to free response questions, *Teaching and Learning in Med.* **5**(2): 107–115.

CASE, S.M., SWANSON, D.B. & RIPKEY, D.R. (1994) Comparison of items in five-options and extended matching format for assessment of diagnostic skills, *Acad. Med.* **71**(suppl): S28–S30.

CASE, S. & SWANSON, D.B. (2002) Constructing written test for the basic and clinical sciences 3rd ed. (National Board of Medical Examiners®, Philadelphia, PA, USA). Web address: http://www.nbme.org/about/itemwriting.asp (last accessed December 2005).

CHAPTER 11

Key Features Test (KF)

Description

The key features test was originally developed by the Medical Council of Canada (MCC) for its licensing examination. It is a clinical scenario-based paper and pencil test. A description of the problem is followed by a limited number of questions, usually two to three, that focus only on *critical, challenging actions or decisions* (Page & Bordage, 1995). Both write-in and short-menu formats can be used in the answer scripts. In the MCC licensing examination, the KF test is implemented along with the more conventional MCQ.

Advantages

- A more valid representation of clinical decision making skills (Page, Bordage, & Allen, 1995)
- Objective marking scheme
- Does not reward unnecessary thoroughness
- KF of cases can be utilized in other examination formats such as MCQ and OSCE

Limitations

- Labor intensive to develop
- Unfamiliarity of examiners and students with the format

Evidence

- High content validity with proper blueprinting (Page & Bordage, 1995)
- 40 problems (approximately 4.1 hour of testing time) are necessary to reach a desired reliability of 0.80 (Page & Bordage, 1995)
- A 15-problem KF examination has a reliability of 0.50 — suitable for medium stakes examination (Hatala & Norman, 2002)

Example

Topic: Seizure in an adult in a life-threatening situation

Key features of this case with suggested answers

KF-1 Generate provisional diagnosis of status epilepticus
KF-2 Secure and maintain cardiorespiratory status
KF-3 Begin initial therapy: normal saline, vitamin B, glucose, diazepam, and phenytoin
KF-4 Elicit history regarding causes: alcohol, medication, drugs, diabetes
KF-5 Order immediate exams: electrolytes, glucose, calcium, arterial blood gas, and brain CT

Mr. "X," a 36-year-old man, is brought to the emergency room in your hospital by ambulance because he fell on the sidewalk unconscious while waiting for the bus. A witness immediately called an ambulance and reported to the ambulance crew that before falling to the ground, he seemed confused, agitated, and was arguing with some invisible person. After falling, he began to twitch for a short while, his face becoming blue, and then he began to have jerky movements all over his body for about a minute. He did not recover consciousness after the episode. During the 10-minute ambulance trip, he presented two other similar episodes, without recovering consciousness, and a third episode that you witnessed on arrival.

His temperature is 37.8°C. He looks neglected and is unconscious. No relatives or friends accompanied Mr. "X."

(*Continued*)

(*Continued*)

Question 1: What is (are) your leading working diagnosis(es) at this point in time? You may list up to two.

Question 2: What is your immediate management at this point in time? List as many things as you feel are appropriate.

Question 3: Ten minutes after arrival, Mr. "X" is still unconscious. The nurse found a telephone number in his wallet that you decide to call immediately. What questions will you ask the person answering the phone — assuming he/she knows the patient? You may select up to six questions. Select option 35 if you think that it is not appropriate to call at this point in time.

Question 4: It has been 15 minutes since Mr. X's arrival. What ancillary exams would you order at this point? You may select as many as you feel appropriate. Select option 35 if you think that ancillary exams are not needed at this point in time.

- Question 1 refers to KF 1
- Question 2 refers to KF 2 and 3
- Question 3 refers to KF 4
- Question 4 refers to KF 5

Adopted with permission from M. Nendaz, MD, MHPE and G. Bordage, MD, PhD.

Recommended practice	Effect and rationale
Use of KF along with MCQ and EMI to test clinical decision making	Assessment of clinical competency in "knows how"
Use of shorter KF test in medium stakes examination	Less laborious; acceptable reliability

References and Further Reading

FARMER, E.A. & PAGE, G. (2005) A practical guide to assessing clinical decision making skills using key feature approach, *Med. Edu.* **39**: 1188–1194.

HATALA, R. & NORMAN, G.R. (2002) Adapting key feature examination for a clinical clerkship, *Med. Edu.* **36**: 160–165.

PAGE, G. & BORDAGE, G. (1995) The Medical Council of Canada's key feature project: A more valid written examination of clinical decision making skills, *Acad. Med.* 70(2): 104–110.

PAGE, G., BORDAGE, G., & ALLEN, T. (1995) Developing key-feature problem and examination to assess clinical decision making skills, *Acad. Med.* 70(3): 194–201.

SECTION 3

Assessment of "Shows How"

CHAPTER 12

Long Case

Common Practice

Involves use of a non-standardized real patient. The candidate is usually assessed on one long case and three to four short cases with oral examination. The candidate may or may not be observed during the examination.

Advantage

- Authenticity: it is argued that the long case provides a unique opportunity to test the physician's tasks and interaction with a real patient

Limitations

- Serious doubts about reliability and consistency
- Poor content validity as only 1–2 cases are tested
- Generalizability across other competencies is poor
- Assessment relies on candidate's *presentation*, representing an assessment of "knows how" — a lower level competency rather than "shows how"

Evidence

- Studies from the American Board of Internal Medicine (ABIM) with two long cases, each examined by two examiners, show that reproducibility of the score is 0.39; meaning 39% of the variability of the score is due to actual performance of students (signal) and the remaining 61% of the variability is due to *errors in measurement* (*noise*) (Noricini, 2002)

- With *one long case*, the coefficient drops to 0.24; thus, scores are composed of three times as much noise as signal (Norcini, 2002)
- The difficulty of the long case is primarily a consequence of the fact that it is a single case examination (Norman, 2003)
- Standardization of questions, patients, and examiners has only a *marginal effect* on improving the reliability (Norman, 2003)
- Increasing the length of examination (without increasing the number of encounters or number of competencies assessed) will not improve validity and reliability significantly
- The long case can be improved significantly by increasing the number of encounters (having more long cases), examiners, or aspects of the competence assessed (Norcini, 2002)
- Even when the reliability of the two case examinations is as high as 0.50, it would require *ten cases and 200 minutes of testing time* to achieve a minimally acceptable level of reliability of 0.85 (Wass *et al.*, 2001)

Recommended practice	Effect and rationale
Abandon single long case in high stakes summative examination	Achieving the desired level of reliability by having 10 long cases and 200 minutes of testing time per candidate is impractical
Use of long case during formative assessment and feedback	Students continue to learn with real patients
Validity and reliability of the long case can be improved by: • Increasing the number of encounters with different patients • Increasing the number of competencies assessed • Having multiple examiners assessing different stations	Will lead to more robust and more generalizable data from the examination

References and Further Reading

NORCINI, J.J. (2002) The death of the long case? *BMJ* **324**(7334): 408–409. Web address: http://www.pubmedcentral.nih.gov/articlerender.fcgi?artid=65539; (last accessed December 2005).

NORMAN, G. (2003) Post graduate assessment — reliability and validity, *Trans J. Coll. Med. S. Afri.* **47**: 71–75.

VLEUTEN, van der C. (2000) Validity of final examination in undergraduate medical training, *BMJ* **321**: 1217–1219.

WASS, V., JONES, R. & VLEUTEN, van der C. (2001) Standardized or real patients to test clinical competence? The long case revisited, *Med. Educ.* **35**: 321–325.

WASS, V., VLEUTEN, van der C, SHATZER, J., & JONES, R. (2001) Assessment of clinical competence, *The Lancet* **357**: 945–949.

CHAPTER 13

Short Case

Common Practice

Involves use of three to four non-standardized real patients with one to two examiners. Usually there is a common marking scheme for all the cases.

Advantages

- Authenticity: provides opportunity for assessment with real patients
- Allows greater sampling than the single long case
- Assessment of clinical examination skills in greater detail
- Good construct validity

Limitations

- Inter-rater reliability is variable for the same examination
- Traditional short cases are less standardized than newer formats such as practical assessment of clinical examination skills (PACES) and OSCE

Evidence

- Short cases are better in discriminating between good and poorly performing students than long cases (Hijazi *et al.*, 2002)

Recommended practice	Effect and rationale
Use standardized multiple short cases; for example PACES or OSCE examination	Better reliability and standardization
Select cases to represent multiple competencies and a variety of clinical problems	Better validity and more generalizable data

References and Further Reading

MRCP (UK) — The clinical examination: practical assessment of clinical examination skills. Web address: http://www.mrcpuk.org/plain/PACES.html (last accessed December 2005).

HIJAZI, Z., PREMADASA, I.G., & MOUSSA, M.A.A.A. (2002) Performances of students in the final examination in paediatrics: importance of short cases, *Arch. Dis. Childhood* **86**: 57–58.

CHAPTER 14

Objective Structured Clinical Examination (OSCE)

Description

OSCE consists of multiple stations (usually 15–20) where each candidate is asked to perform a defined task such as taking a focused history or performing a focused examination of a particular system. A standardized marking scheme specific for each case is used.

Advantages

- An effective alternative to unstructured short cases
- Allows wider sampling and standardization of cases
- Greater reliability of marking

Limitations

- Validity is compromised if a complex skill, in the pursuit of higher reliability, is fragmented into multiple minor tasks (Wass, 2001)
- Assessment of communication, and especially attitudes, is difficult, as these skills are case-specific and have poor generalizability. For example, to assess empathy reliably, as many as 37 cases might be required (Colliver *et al.*, 1998)
- OSCE relies on task-specific checklists which assumes that physician-patient interactions can be described as a list of actions (Smee, 2003)
- Labor intensive and expensive

Evidence

- An OSCE with 14–18 stations is recommended so as to obtain a reliable measure of performance (ACGME, 2001)
- There is little difference between marking by the patient or by the examiner (van der Vleuten, 1990)
- Global rating produces equivalent results as compared to checklist (Norman, 2003) — a fact that works *in favor* of test developers and examiners
- Reliability during OSCE is more of a function of the number of stations and competence tested rather than the length of stations (Newble & Swanson, 1988). An OSCE examination comprising 6 stations of 20 minutes' length (2 hours testing time) will produce *less reliable* results compared to 16 stations each lasting 7.5 minutes (equivalent 2 hours of testing time)
- If examiner availability is an issue, more could be gained by having one examiner per station and increasing the number of stations than having two examiners per station and halving the number of stations (Newble & Swanson, 1988)

Example

Communication and counselling OSCE
(Adopted with permission from Drs Marion Aw, Low Poh Sim, and Daniel Goh, Department of Paediatrics, Yong Loo Lin School of Medicine, National University of Singapore, Singapore.)

Introduction to candidates

This is a ten (10) minute patient instruction station.
Read the scenario carefully.
(A clean placebo device is provided for your use)

Scenario

Mandy is a 7-year-old girl with mild persistent asthma diagnosed one year ago. She has just been admitted to hospital following an exacerbation of asthma.

She is on salbutamol and beclomethasone Meter Dose Inhaler (MDI with spacer device).

(*Continued*)

(*Continued*)

Mandy's mother requests you to review the MDI technique with her, as she is concerned that she could have been doing it "wrong." On questioning, you realize that Mandy's mother has stopped using the beclomethasone inhaler because it is not helping to relieve her symptoms.

Mandy's mother has asked for a doctor to show her how to use the inhaler so that she can help Mandy use it.

Task: You, as her doctor today, are expected to check on the technique of inhaler use and give appropriate instructions to the mother. Enter the room and speak to her.

Instructions to examiners

Key features of OSCE

The candidate is expected to communicate clear and precise instructions on:

- The correct technique of using the MDI with a spacer device
- The role of beclomethasone MDI as a preventer of asthma and the importance of using it regularly

Note

- One nurse will role-play as Mandy's mother
- The examiner is to assess the candidate's performance during the consultation
- The candidate will not score better than "*borderline fail*" in overall performance if he/she is unable to teach the right technique

Instructions to standardised patient: patient's script

Background for simulated patient

Mandy is a 7-year-old who developed asthma about one year ago. She has mild to moderate persistent asthma which is often precipitated by upper respiratory tract infection.

(*Continued*)

(*Continued*)

She was initially treated with salbutamol MDI but beclomethasone MDI was added later on as the symptoms continued to persist.

This is Mandy's first hospitalization. Mandy's mother has not been giving the medication to her regularly for the past two weeks. In particular, she feels that there has been no improvement when using the brown (beclomethasone MDI) inhaler.

Mandy's mother also wants to know how to recognize whether the medication in the MDI has run out.

Starting the role play

Lead-in statement: "Doctor, I was wondering if you could go through with me how to use this inhaler. I have been using it as instructed by the doctor, yet Mandy did not improve. Maybe I got the technique wrong."

Pause for the candidate to respond.

(After 1 min) If the doctor does not offer to observe you demonstrate the use of the MDI, prompt by saying, "Would you like me to show you how I've been teaching my daughter how to use the inhaler?"

(After 5 min) If the doctor has not demonstrated to you how to use the inhaler or has asked you to demonstrate to him/her before showing you first, prompt by saying, "Doctor, why don't you show me exactly what you mean?"

(After 7 min) If the doctor has not asked you to demonstrate the correct usage, prompt by asking, "Doctor, why don't I show you again to make sure that I've got it right?"

Next statement "How will I tell if the medication in the MDI has run out?"

Candidate to demonstrate how to test MDI by shaking the MDI and actuating a dose.

Sample of answer/reference material

Steps in spacer with mask usage:

- Remove the cover from the inhaler mouth-piece and shake the MDI canister
- Fit the inhaler mouth-piece to the spacer device
- Ensure a tight seal of the lips over the device
- Place canister mouth piece at the other end of the spacer device and press the canister of the inhaler down firmly to release the medicine
- Inhale and exhale with mouth over the spacer device for about 10 times
- Repeat the steps for second puff, and as many puffs as instructed

Equipment and resources

- Standardized patient
- Placebo inhaler: salbutamol and beclomethasone (2 sets per station)
- Spacer device: (2 sets per station)
- Disinfectant/cleaning provisions

Rating Checklist

	Key points	Performed competently	Performed but NOT fully competent	Not performed or incompetent
A	**Communication and Rapport**			
	Candidate greets the mother & introduces self	1	0.5	0
	Sensitive to parent's concern	1	0.5	0
B	**Problem Identification**			
	Notes that the "patient's" PRN use of the beclomethasone MDI is wrong	1	—	0
	Asks parent to demonstrate use of MDI	2	1*	0
	Detects parent's wrong technique of using MDI	1	—	0
C	**Demonstration and Patient Education**			
	Demonstrates use of MDI to mother	2	1*	0
	Removes the cover from inhaler and shakes the inhaler	1	—	0
	Fits the inhaler to the spacer	1	—	0
	Demonstrates a tight seal of the lips over the device	1	—	0
	Presses the canister of the inhaler down firmly to release the medicine	1	—	0
	Breathes in and out normally several times	1	—	0
	Emphasizes beclomethasone as an important treatment for the patient	2	1	0
	Asks mother to demonstrate again the use of the MDI	2	1*	0
	Demonstrates how to recognize that MDI has run out of medication	1	—	0
D	**Closing**			
	Asks the mother about her understanding	2	1	0

* With prompting.

Recommended practice	Effect and rationale
An OSCE should have at least 14–18 stations	Required to achieve acceptable level of reliability
Use of global rating scale and examiner training	Global rating scale is as good as more labor intensive check-list based scoring
Use of patients as raters	Reduces need for expert examiners Produces equivalent results

Tips on Writing OSCE

- Develop a case blueprint for entire examination
- Focus on the important physician's tasks
- Spend more energy and efforts in increasing the number of stations and less on standardizing the checklist or marking scheme
- If examiner availability is an issue, consider using the standardized patient as a marker
- Do not separate artificially the content and the process; for most tasks these two are inseparable

References and Further Reading

ACGME Outcome Project. Accreditation Council For Graduate Medical Education (ACGME) and American Board Of Medical Specialist (ABMS). (2001) Toolbox of assessment methods, version 1.1. Web address www.acgme.org/Outcome/assess/Toolbox.pdf (last accessed December 2005).

COLLIVER, J.A., WILLIS, M.S., ROBBS, R.S., COHEN, D.S., & SWARTZ, M.H. (1998) Assessment of empathy in a standardized-patient examination, *Teaching and Learning in Med.* **10**: 8–11.

NEWBLE, D. & SWANSON, D.B. (1988) Psychometric characteristics of the objective structured clinical test, *Med. Edu.* **22**(4): 325–334.

NORMAN, G. (2003) Post graduate assessment — reliability and validity, *Trans. J. Coll. Med. S. Afri.* **47**: 71–75.

SMEE, S. (2003) Skill based assessment, *BMJ* **326**: 703–706. Web address: http://bmj.bmjjournals.com/cgi/reprint/326/7391/703 (last accessed December 2005).

SECTION 4

Assessment of "Does"

CHAPTER 15

Mini-Clinical Evaluation Exercise (Mini-CEX)

Description

Mini-clinical evaluation exercise is a rating scale developed by the American Board of Internal Medicine (ABIM) in the 1990s to assess six core competencies of residents. These are:

- medical interviewing skills
- physical examination skills
- humanistic qualities/professionalism
- clinical judgment
- counselling skills
- organization and efficiency

There is another category for overall clinical competency (Norcini, 1995).

Each competency is rated from 1 to 9 (1–3 unsatisfactory, 4–6 satisfactory, 7–9 superior). Each competency is defined with an anchored statement. For example, an expected performance in physical examination skill is "follows efficient, logical sequence; balances screening/diagnostic steps for problem; informs patient; sensitive to patient's comfort, modesty."

For each encounter, the evaluator records the complexity of the patient's problem (low, moderate, high); type of visit (new or return); setting (ward, emergency room, clinic, or ICU); focus of the visit (data gathering, diagnosis, therapy, or counselling); time spent observing the encounter; and time spent in giving feedback.

Each encounter lasts for about 15–25 minutes, including the time spent on the feedback given to the trainee. The reliability improves with greater numbers of observed encounters and 4–6 encounters are required to reach an acceptable reliability. Once completed, the mini-CEX becomes an integral part of the trainee's training records.

Mini-CEX is now a requirement of trainee evaluation in the National Health Service (NHS), UK (Modernising Medical Career, MMC, NHS). The MMC website contains a variety of mini-CEX resources, including orientation video and forms.

Advantages

- Direct observation of candidate performance
- Allows global evaluation of performance
- Good inter-rater reliability
- Practical and easy to use
- Possible to customize to local contexts and needs

Limitations

- Relatively new and unfamiliar
- Faculty training is needed to improve reliability
- It is not possible to assess all aspects of competencies through a single encounter

Evidence

- Mini-CEX is helpful in discriminating different levels of performance (Holmboe, 2003)
- Its reliability and reproducibility is 0.73 and above (Norcini, 2003)
- Reliability improves with greater number of encounters and at least 4–6 encounters are needed to reach acceptable reliability (Norcini, 2003)
- Mini-CEX is user- and time-friendly (Kogan, 2002)
- Mini-CEX is highly acceptable to both faculty and trainee (Kogan, 2002)

Sample Mini-CEX Data Collection Form

Evaluator: **Date:** **Student:**

Setting: ☐ OPD ☐ In-patient ☐ ED ☐ Other

Patient: ☐ Age Sex: M/F ☐ New ☐ Follow-up

Complexity: ☐ Low ☐ Moderate ☐ High

Focus ☐ Data Gathering ☐ Diagnosis ☐ Therapy ☐ Counselling

1. **Medical Interviewing Skills** [0 Not observed]
   1 2 3 4 5 6 7 8 9
   Unsatisfactory Satisfactory Superior
2. **Physical Examination Skills** [0 Not observed]
   1 2 3 4 5 6 7 8 9
   Unsatisfactory Satisfactory Superior
3. **Humanistic Qualification/Professionalism** [0 Not observed]
   1 2 3 4 5 6 7 8 9
   Unsatisfactory Satisfactory Superior
4. **Clinical Judgment** [0 Not observed]
   1 2 3 4 5 6 7 8 9
   Unsatisfactory Satisfactory Superior
5. **Counselling Skills** [0 Not observed]
   1 2 3 4 5 6 7 8 9
   Unsatisfactory Satisfactory Superior
6. **Organizational Efficiency** [0 Not observed]
   1 2 3 4 5 6 7 8 9
   Unsatisfactory Satisfactory Superior
7. **Overall Clinical Competency** [0 Not observed]
   1 2 3 4 5 6 7 8 9
   Unsatisfactory Satisfactory Superior

Mini-CEX time: observing: .... min Providing Feedback: ....min

Evaluator's Satisfaction with mini-CEX

Low 1 2 3 4 5 6 7 8 9 High

Student's Satisfaction with mini-CEX

Low 1 2 3 4 5 6 7 8 9 High

Comments:

Adapted from: American Board of Internal Medicine. PA. USA. Web address: www.abim.org.

Suggested Uses

- Direct observation of student's performance with real patients
- Feedback and formative assessment to the students
- Competency assessment

References and Further Reading

HOLMBOE, E.S., HUOT, S., CHUNG, J., NORCINI, J., & HAWKINS, R.E. (2003) Construct validity of the mini-clinical evaluation exercise (mini-CEX), *Acad. Med.* 78(8): 826–830. Web address: http://www.academicmedicine.org/cgi/content/full/78/8/826 (last accessed December 2005).

KOGAN, J.R., BELLINI, L.M., & SHEA, J.A. (2002) Implementation of the mini-CEX to evaluate medical students' clinical skills, *Acad. Med.* 77(11): 1156–1157.

MODERNISING MEDICAL CAREER. Mini-CEX (Clinical Evaluation Exercise), National Health Service. Web address: http://www.mmc.nhs.uk/pages/assessment/minicex (last accessed December 2005).

NORCINI, J.J., BLANK, L.L., ARNOLD, G.K., & KIMBALL, H.R. (1995) Mini-CEX (clinical evaluation exercise) A preliminary investigations, *Ann. Inter. Med.* **123**(10): 795–799. Web address: http://www.annals.org/cgi/content/full/123/10/795 (last accessed December 2005).

NORCINI, J.J., BLANK, L.L., DUFFY, F.D., & FORTNA, G.S. (2003) The mini-CEX: a method for assessing clinical skills, *Ann. Inter. Med.* **138**(6): 476–481. Web address: http://www.annals.org/cgi/reprint/138/6/476 (last accessed December 2005).

CHAPTER 16

Direct Observation of Procedural Skills (DOPS)

Description

Direct Observation of Procedural Skills (DOPS) is a structured rating scale for assessing and providing feedback on practical procedures. DOPS is similar to mini-CEX except that the domains of interest are related to practical procedures.

Depending on the design of the form, the competencies that are commonly assessed include general knowledge about the procedure, informed consent, pre-procedure preparation, analgesia/sedation, technical ability, aseptic technique, post-procedure management, and counselling and communication. In a given encounter, it may not be possible to observe and assess all the domains of interest. Nevertheless, with multiple encounters, with different patients, and with varied procedures it is possible to gather reasonable evidence about a student's or a trainee's global competency in technical skills.

Each encounter lasts for about 15–25 minutes, including the time spent on the feedback given to the student. The reliability improves with greater numbers of observed encounters and it needs 4–6 encounters to reach an acceptable reliability.

Like the mini-CEX, DOPS is now a training requirement for trainees under the National Health Service (NHS), UK. NHS maintains a website (www.mmc.nhs.uk/pages/assessment/DOPS) for trainees and assessors on DOPS. The website includes a video and other relevant resources.

Advantages

- Direct observation of procedural skills
- Allows global evaluation
- Practical and easy to use
- Possible to customize to local contexts and needs

Limitations

- Relatively new and unfamiliar
- Faculty training is needed
- It is not possible to assess all aspects of competencies through a single encounter
- If a procedure is technical in nature, it may be necessary to have an expert observer or assessor

Sample DOPS Data Collection Form

Evaluator: **Date:** **Student:**

Setting: ☐ OPD ☐ In-patient ☐ ED ☐ OT ☐ Other

Patient: Age Sex: M/F ☐ New ☐ Follow-up

Complexity: ☐ Low ☐ Moderate ☐ High

Name of the Procedure: [ ]

1. **Demonstrate understanding of indications, relevant anatomy, technique of procedures** [0 Not observed/unable to comment]
   1 2 3 (Unsatisfactory) 4 5 6 (Satisfactory) 7 8 9 (Superior)
2. **Obtain informed consent** [0 Not observed/unable to comment]
   1 2 3 (Unsatisfactory) 4 5 6 (Satisfactory) 7 8 9 (Superior)
3. **Demonstrate appropriate preparation; pre-procedure** [0 Not observed/unable to comment]
   1 2 3 (Unsatisfactory) 4 5 6 (Satisfactory) 7 8 9 (Superior)
4. **Appropriate analgesia/safe sedation** [0 Not observed/unable to comment]
   1 2 3 (Unsatisfactory) 4 5 6 (Satisfactory) 7 8 9 (Superior)
5. **Technical ability** [0 Not observed/unable to comment]
   1 2 3 (Unsatisfactory) 4 5 6 (Satisfactory) 7 8 9 (Superior)
6. **Aseptic technique** [0 Not observed/unable to comment]
   1 2 3 (Unsatisfactory) 4 5 6 (Satisfactory) 7 8 9 (Superior)
7. **Seek help where appropriate** [0 Not observed/unable to comment]
   1 2 3 (Unsatisfactory) 4 5 6 (Satisfactory) 7 8 9 (Superior)
8. **Post procedure management** [0 Not observed/unable to comment]
   1 2 3 (Unsatisfactory) 4 5 6 (Satisfactory) 7 8 9 (Superior)
9. **Communication skills** [0 Not observed/unable to comment]
   1 2 3 (Unsatisfactory) 4 5 6 (Satisfactory) 7 8 9 (Superior)
10. **Consideration of patient/professionalism** [0 Not observed/unable to comment]
    1 2 3 (Unsatisfactory) 4 5 6 (Satisfactory) 7 8 9 (Superior)

11. **Overall ability to perform the procedure** [0 Not observed/unable to comment]

1 2 3	4 5 6	7 8 9
Unsatisfactory	Satisfactory	Superior

DOPS time: Observing: ....min Providing Feedback: .... min

Evaluator's Satisfaction

Low 1 2 3 4 5 6 7 8 9 High

Resident's Satisfaction

Low 1 2 3 4 5 6 7 8 9 High

Comments:

Adopted from: National Health Service Modernising Medical Career (MMC); UK. Web address: http://www.mmc.nhs.uk/pages/assessment/dops.

Suggested Uses

- Direct observation and assessment of procedural and practical skills in real situations
- Feedback and formative assessment to the students and trainees
- Competency assessment

References and Further Reading

MODERNISING MEDICAL CAREER. DOPS (Direct Observation of Procedural Skills). National Health Service. Web address: http://www.mmc.nhs.uk/pages/assessment/dops; (last accessed December 2005).

CHAPTER 17

Clinical Work Sampling (CWS)

Description

Clinical Work Sampling (CWS) is an in-trainee evaluation method. Like the mini-CEX and DOPS, the CWS addresses the issue of system and rater biases by collecting data on observed behavior at the time of actual performance and by using multiple observers and occasions. Like the mini-CEX and DOPS, there is an opportunity to provide feedback to the student and trainee.

The design of the form takes into account the context of patient encounters, and different forms are used in different situations. Thus, Admission Rating Forms collect data on communication skills, physical examination skills, diagnostic acumen, management skills, and global performance. Patient Rating Forms capture data on four domains: communication skills, collaboration skills, health advocacy skills, and professionalism (Turnbull *et al.*, 2000).

Advantages

- Direct observation of performance
- Authentic as the assessment takes place during work
- Multiple data sources
- Takes into account different clinical situations
- Includes data from patients

Limitations

- Relatively new and less well studied
- Difficult to obtain data from patients

Items Evaluated in Clinical Work Sampling (CWS)

Admission Rating Form
Diagnostic/therapeutic plan
Differential diagnosis
Physical examination
Communication skills (written and verbal)
Overall impression
Ward Rating Form
Diagnostic/therapeutic plan
Communication skills
Consultation skills
Management of resources
Health advocacy skills
Interpersonal skills
Fund of knowledge
Overall impression
Multidisciplinary Team Rating Form
Diagnostic/therapeutic plan
Communication skills
Consultation skills
Management of resources
Discharge planning
Interpersonal skills
Overall impression
Patient Rating Form (content domains; administered through interview)
Communication skills
Collaboration skills
Health advocacy skills
Professionalism
Overall impression

Rating scale used: 1 = satisfactory; 2 = meets expectations; 3 = good; 4 = very good; and 5 = excellent.

Adapted from: TURNBULL, J., MACFADYEN, J., BARNEVELD, C. VAN, & NORMAN, G. (2000) Clinical work sampling: a new approach to the problem of in-training evaluation, *J. Gen. Inter. Med.* 15: 556–561. Used with authors' permission.

Suggested Uses

- Direct observation of performance in real clinical situations
- Feedback and formative assessment to students and trainees
- Competency assessment

References and Further Reading

TURNBULL, J., MACFADYEN, J., BARNEVELD, C. VAN, & NORMAN, G. (2000) Clinical work sampling a new approach to the problem of in-training evaluation, *J. Gen. Inter. Med.* 15: 556–561.

CHAPTER 18
Checklist

Description

Checklists are commonly used in assessments to capture an observed behavior or action of a student. Generally, rating is by a five to seven point Likert scale (e.g. agree, somewhat agree, neutral, somewhat disagree, disagree). Checklists are usually used at the end of clinical rotations.

Advantages

- Easy to develop
- Captures actual action and performed behavior

Limitations

- Often casually developed and implemented
- Validity depends on the representativeness of items on checklist for the expected and desired competency
- Inter-rater disagreement is a problem
- Evaluation based on a "single global rating scale completed at infrequent intervals by a supervisor" has poor reliability and is prone to random and systemic rater biases (Turnbull *et al.*, 2000)

Evidence

- Content validity (importance of items in the checklist) can be improved by getting the agreement of experts (Nørgaard, Ringsted, & Dolmans, 2004)

- Inter-rater agreement can be improved by having anchored statements and faculty training by analysis of video-taped performance of candidates (Holmboe, Hawkins & Houts, 2004)

Recommended practice	Effect and rationale
In-house, locally developed checklists need to be researched before being used for summative assessment	Necessary for checklist validation
For summative assessment, it is important to use *pre-validated* checklists	Important for medium to high stakes examinations
Use of anchored checklists and faculty training	Better description of behaviour and faculty training result in better reliability
Alternatives: 360-degree evaluation with multiple raters and pre-validated checklist	Better objective data, use of pre-validated instruments

Example

A validated checklist to assess ward round performance

Setting the stage for rounds: Introduction and preparation
1. Clarifies who will participate. Clarifies whether team discussion should take place prior to patient round
2. Clarifies any organizational issues of importance (e.g. occupancy rate, expected new admission, expected discharges, and staff shortage)
The patient round/consultation with patients
3. Reviews hospital course of each patient through chart review
4. Evaluates new lab results, X-rays, medications, etc. Makes relevant follow-up and adjustments
5. Performs an effective consultation with each patient, including interview, examination, and information given by the nurse-team
6. Discusses medical issues with nurse-team, taking into consideration existing patient management plans and necessary adjustments
7. Summarizes the hospital course with the patient and plans for further investigations, treatment and discharge. Specifies issues, which will be decided on later, including when and how these decisions will be made. Ensures patient's understanding and agreement of the plans
After round: Closing the ward round
8. Summarizes the ward round and the plans, including timelines and consultations or further discussions that will take place
9. Summarizes and seeks consensus on agreements with the team on these plans
10. Evaluates the ward round with nurse team

NØRGAARD, K., RINGSTED, C., & DOLMANS, D. (2004) Validation of a checklist to assess ward round performance in internal medicine, *Med. Edu.* **38**: 700–707. Used with permission.

References and Further Reading

HOLMBOE, E.S., HAWKINS, R.E., & HUOT, S.J. (2004) Effects of training in direct observation of medical residents' clinical competence: a randomized trial, *Ann. Inter. Med.* **140**(11): 874–881. Web address http://www.annals.org/cgi/reprint/140/11/874.pdf (last accessed December 2005).

NØRGAARD, K., RINGSTED, C., & DOLMANS, D. (2004) Validation of a checklist to assess ward round performance in internal medicine, *Med. Edu.* **38**: 700–707.

TURNBULL, J., MACFADYEN, J., BARNEVELD VAN, C., & NORMAN, G. (2000) Clinical work sampling: a new approach to the problem of in-training evaluation, *J. Gen. Inter. Med.* **15**: 556–561.

CHAPTER 19

360-Degree Evaluation

Description

A 360-degree evaluation consists of measurement tools completed by multiple individuals in a person's sphere of influence (ACGME, 2000). Usually, it assesses how frequently a behavior or an action is performed by a candidate using a rating scale (e.g. 1 = frequently, 5 = never). The observation is done by many different individuals, and generally includes the supervising physicians, peers and nurses.

The domain of competency assessed by a 360-degree evaluation is generally restricted to aspects of observable behavior such as communication skills, interpersonal relationship, and others.

360-degree evaluation is also known as Multi Source Feedback (MSF).

Advantages

- Assessment of actual action and behavior
- Assessment by multiple observers
- Provides evidence, as opposed to impression, about individual
- Highly valued as a developmental tool

Limitations

- Limited research regarding psychometric qualities of 360-degree evaluation
- Evaluators might hesitate to provide accurate rating in poorly performing candidates

- Cumbersome data collection and analysis from a large number of raters

Evidence

- A high degree of reproducibility (0.90) reported in other professional education (ACGME, 2001)
- Reproducibility is better with nurse raters as compared to faculty raters (ACGME, 2001)

Suggested Use

- Assessment of Behavior

Recommended practice	Effect and rationale
Implementation and monitoring of 360-degree evaluation tool during ward posting	Assessment of actual performance of students in authentic setting
Use 360-degree evaluation to assess "softer" qualities such as collegiality, approachability, communication, and professional behavior	These qualities are difficult to assess using other existing tools

A Sample 360-Degree (Multi-Source Feedback) Evaluation Form

This form is not intended to be used for assessment of knowledge and practical skills.

1. **Attitude to staff: Respects and values contribution of other members of the team**
   1 2 3 4 5 6 7 8 9
   Unsatisfactory Satisfactory Superior
2. **Attitudes to patients: Respects the rights, choices, beliefs, and confidentiality of patients**
   1 2 3 4 5 6 7 8 9
   Unsatisfactory Satisfactory Superior
3. **Reliability and punctuality**
   1 2 3 4 5 6 7 8 9
   Unsatisfactory Satisfactory Superior
4. **Communication skills: Communicates effectively with patients and family**
   1 2 3 4 5 6 7 8 9
   Unsatisfactory Satisfactory Superior
5. **Communication skills: Communicates effectively with healthcare professionals**
   1 2 3 4 5 6 7 8 9
   Unsatisfactory Satisfactory Superior
6. **Team player skills: Supportive and accepts appropriate responsibility; approachable**
   1 2 3 4 5 6 7 8 9
   Unsatisfactory Satisfactory Superior
7. **Leadership skills: Takes responsibility of own actions and actions of the team**
   1 2 3 4 5 6 7 8 9
   Unsatisfactory Satisfactory Superior
8. **Overall professional competency**
   1 2 3 4 5 6 7 8 9
   Unsatisfactory Satisfactory Superior

Comments:

Adapted from: National Health Service Modernising Medical Career (MMC); UK. Web address: http://www.mmc.nhs.uk/pages/assessment/msf.

References and Further Reading

ACGME Outcome Project. Accreditation Council For Graduate Medical Education (ACGME) & American Board Of Medical Specialist (ABMS). (2001) Toolbox of assessment methods, version 1.1. Web address www.acgme.org/Outcome/assess/Toolbox.pdf (last accessed December 2005).

RAKSHA, J., LING, F.W., & JAEGER, J. (2004) Assessment of a 360-degree instrument to evaluate residents' competency in interpersonal and communication skills, *Acad. Med.* 79: 458–463.

CHAPTER 20

Log Book

Description

The candidate or student keeps a record of the patients seen or procedures performed either in a book or in a computer. The program may or may not have a defined target (e.g. number of procedures to be performed, types and number of cases to be seen) for the candidate.

Advantages

- Documents the range of patient care and learning experiences of students
- Very useful in focusing students on important objectives that must be fulfilled within a specified period of time (Blake, 2001)
- Ensures uniformity of students' experience as students may have very different learning experiences even in seemingly similar rotations

Limitations

- Accuracy of students' reporting and faculty grading is difficult to ascertain
- Minimum number of procedures to be performed and cases to be seen is often set arbitrarily and is not validated against performance in the future (ACGME, 2001)
- The number of procedures performed and patients seen does not necessarily correlate with competence achieved (ACGME, 2001)
- Unlike portfolios, there is no scope for personal goal settings and reflection

Recommended practice	Effect and rationale
Use of log book during ward posting	Assessment of actual experience of students in authentic settings
Develop the target of achievement (e.g. number of cases seen, procedures performed) with rigorous expert consensus	Required for validation of actual performance in future

References and Further Reading

ACGME Outcome Project. Toolbox for Assessment Methods. Accreditation Council for Graduate Medical Education (ACGME) and American Board of Medical Specialist (ABMS). Version 1.1. 2000. Web address: http://www.acgme.org/Outcome/assess/Toolbox.pdf (last accessed December 2005).

BLAKE, K. (2001) The daily grind — use of log books and portfolios for documenting undergraduates activities, *Med. Edu.* 35: 1097–1098.

CHAPTER 21

Portfolio

Description

A portfolio is a collection of one's professional and personal goals, achievements, and methods of achieving these goals (Amin and Khoo, 2003). It may contain items such as one's best essays, written or research projects, log books, letter of reflection and evidence of professional growth, to support individual accomplishment and progression (Friedman *et al.*, 2001).

Advantages

- Collects evidence of actual performance in the "Does" level in a longitudinal manner
- Highly valued as a formative assessment and feedback tool

Limitations

- Time consuming on the part of faculty and students to maintain a detailed portfolio
- Difficult to mark and standardize
- Difficult to decide on a pass/fail cut-off

Evidence

- Validity of the portfolio is largely dependent on the extent items contained in the portfolio actually demonstrate mastery of expected learning (ACGME, 2000)

- Inter-rater agreement of marking portfolio is reported to be 0.60 to 0.70 (Le Mahier *et al.*, 1993 cited by Friedman *et al.*, 2001)
- The amount of text written in the portfolio corresponds to the final grade ($p < 0.001$; $F = 4.2$) (Lonka *et al.*, 2001)
- Experience from Singapore with a Family Medicine training program shows that a one-page portfolio helps trainees to cover a broad range of topics

Recommended practice	Effect and rationale
Use portfolio as a part of formative assessment	Support of student learning

References and Further Reading

ACGME Outcome Project. Toolbox for Assessment Methods. Accreditation Council for Graduate Medical Education (ACGME) and American Board of Medical Specialist (ABMS). Version 1.1. 2000. Web address: http://www.acgme.org/Outcome/assess/Toolbox.pdf (last accessed December 2005).

AMIN, Z. & KHOO, H.E. (2003) *Basics in Medical Education* (World Scientific Publishing Company, Singapore).

FRIEDMAN-BEN DAVID, M., DAVIS M.H., HARDEN, R.M., HOWIE, P.W., KER, J., & PIPPERD, M.J. (2001) Portfolio as a method of student assessment, AMEE Education Guide 24 (Association of Medical Education in Europe, Dundee, UK).

LIM, J., CHAN, N., & CHEONG, P. (1998) Experience with portfolio-based learning in family medicine for Master of Medicine degree, *Sing. Med. J.* 39: 543–546. Web address: http://www.sma.org.sg/smj/3912/articles/3912a2.html (last accessed December 2005).

LONKA, K., SLOTTE, V., HALTTUNEN, K. T., TIITINEN, A., VAARA, L., & PAAOVONEN, J. (2001) Portfolios as a learning tool in obstetrics and gynaecology undergraduate training, *Med. Edu.* 35(12): 1125–1130.

APPENDIX A
Summary of Recommendations

Recommendations for Better Practice

- Assessment should be designed prospectively along with learning outcomes
- Assessment methods must provide valid and usable data
- Assessment methods must yield reliable and generalizable data
- Assessment should be driven by the purpose in mind
- Multiple assessment instruments targeting all levels in Miller's pyramid are necessary to capture reasonable breadth of competency
- Content validity is best achieved by a proper blueprint of learning outcomes
- Students need to be tested with multiple cases and scenarios to achieve an acceptable degree of reliability
- Standard of the examination should be based on criterion-based referencing

A Proposed Backbone of Assessment for Undergraduate Medical Curriculum

Several recurring themes emerge from the previous discussion and analysis of psychometric and other properties assessment methods.

- Multiple assessment methods are necessary to capture all or most aspects of clinical competency and any single method is not sufficient to do the job
- Validity of the clinical assessment is a matter of the entire examination and not just the property of one single assessment method
- Multiple sampling strategy is essential to have improved reliability and validity
- Practical issues and efficiency should be considered in selecting a test method
- Compromise is invariable; informed decision is the key

Based on all these factors and the level of readiness in many medical schools, we propose the following schema for medium to high stakes assessment. We believe it is a reasonably informed compromise between the overarching need of maintaining a high degree of validity and reliability and the practicality of administering such tests.

We propose that this schema of assessment should constitute the *backbone of the assessment*. This can be supplemented, if necessary, with other forms of occasional assessment methods to cater to specific needs of a given situation.

For knowledge, concepts, application of knowledge ("knows" and "knows how")

- Preferred: context-based MCQ, extended matching item (EMI), short answer questions
- Not recommended: long essay question, viva, true-false type MCQ
- Promising: key feature test

For "shows how"

- Preferred: multi-station objective structured objective examination (OSCE)
- Alternatives: multiple short cases with structured marking scheme and multiple examiners
- Not recommended: single long case, traditional viva

For performance-based assessment ("does")

- Preferred: mini-CEX, DOPS (for procedural skills), 360-degree evaluation
- Alternatives: portfolio, log-book, clinical work sampling
- Not recommended: retrospective end of posting assessment with single assessor

APPENDIX B

Annotated References and Further Reading

*Articles of special interest

**Articles of outstanding interest

2006 Step 1 Content description and sample test materials. (2005) Published by the Federation of State Medical Boards of the United States, Inc. and the National Board of Medical Examiners® (NBME®). Web address: http://www.usmle.org/step1/default.htm.

**ACGME Outcome Project. Accreditation Council for Graduate Medical Education (ACGME) & American Board of Medical Specialist (ABMS). (2001) Toolbox of assessment methods, version 1.1. Web address www.acgme.org/Outcome/assess/Toolbox.pdf.

(A downloadable guide of assessment methods used predominantly during on-the-job assessment of residents. Includes brief psychometric characteristics and references.)

AMIN, Z. & KHOO, H.E. (2003) *Basics in Medical Education* (World Scientific Publishing Company, Singapore, 2003). Web address: http://www.worldscibooks.com/medsci/5140.html.

(An easy-to-read introduction to medical education for medical teachers; contains several chapters on broad overview of assessment. Available from the publisher and all major online bookstores.)

BEULLEN, J., STRUVF, E., & DAMME, B.V. (2005) Do extended matching multiple choice questions measure clinical reasoning? *Med. Edu.* **39**(4): 410–415.

BLAKE, K. (2001) The daily grind — use of log books and portfolios for documenting undergraduate activities, *Med. Edu.* **35** 1097–1098.

CAMPBELL, L.M. (1995) Improving oral examination, *BMJ* **311**: 1572–1573.

CASE, S.M. & SWANSON, D.B. (1993) Extended matching items: a practical alternative to free response questions, *Teaching and Learning in Med.* **5**(2): 107–115.

CASE, S.M., SWANSON, D.B., & RIPKEY, D.R. (1994) Comparison of items in five-options and extended matching format for assessment of diagnostic skills, *Acad. Med.* **71**(suppl): S28–S30.

(Research article confirming the value of EMI.)

**CASE, S. & SWANSON, D.B. (2002) Constructing written test for the basic and clinical sciences, 3rd ed. (National Board of Medical Examiners®,

Philadelphia, PA, USA). Web address: http://www.nbme.org/about/itemwriting.asp.

(A definitive guide on MCQ and EMI by two eminent educationists. A must read for anyone involved in writing MCQ. It is downloadable in full from the NBME® website.)

CASHIN, W.E. (1987) Improving essay tests. Idea Paper No. 17, Center for Faculty Evaluation and Development. Kansas State University, Kansas, USA. Web address: http://www.idea.ksu.edu/papers/Idea_Paper_17.pdf.

COLLIVER, J.A., WILLIS, M.S., ROBBS, R.S., COHEN, D.S., & SWARTZ, M.H. (1998) Assessment of empathy in a standardized-patient examination, *Teaching and Learning in Med.* **10**: 8–11.

*DAY, S.C., NORCINI, J.J., DISERENS, D., *et al.* (1990) The validity of an essay test of clinical judgment, *Acad. Med.* **65**(9): S39–S40.

EPSTEIN, R.M. & HUNDERT, E.M. (2002) Defining and assessing clinical competence, *JAMA* **387: 226–235.

(An excellent review article on clinical competence. Proposes a broader definition of clinical competence and an elaborate schema of competencies necessary.)

ELSTEIN, A.S., SHULMAN, L.S., & SPRAFKA, S.A. (1978) *Medical Problem-solving: An Analysis of Clinical Reasoning* (Harvard University Press, Cambridge, MA, USA).

(An early book on clinical decision making, diagnostic reasoning.)

*FARMER, E.A. & PAGE, G. (2005) A practical guide to assessing clinical decision making skills using key feature approach, *Med. Edu.* **39**: 1188–1194.

*FRIEDMAN BEN-DAVID, M. (2000) Standard setting in student assessment, AMEE Education Guide 18 (Association for Medical Education in Europe, Dundee, UK).

(Part of a series of Guide on Medical Education. Include step-by-step procedures of setting standard.)

*FRIEDMAN BEN DAVID, M., DAVIS, M.H., HARDEN, R.M., HOWIE, P.W., KER, J., & PIPPERD, M.J. (2001) Portfolio as a method of student assessment, AMEE Education Guide 24 (Association of Medical Education in Europe, Dundee, UK).

(Elaborate discussion on educational underpinnings, usefulness, uses and limitations of portfolio as a summative instrument. An earlier guide,

Portfolio Learning in Medical Education, discusses value of portfolio as a learning tool.)

RAKSHA, J., LING, F.W., & JAEGER, J. (2004) Assessment of a 360-degree instrument to evaluate residents' competency in interpersonal and communication skills, *Acad. Med.* **79**: 458–463.

JOZEFOWICZ, R.F., KOEPPEN, B.M., CASE, S., GALBRAITH, R., SWANSON, D., & GLEW, R.H. (2002). The quality of in-house examination, *Acad. Med.* 77(2): 156–161.

(A research conducted among the leading US medical schools establishes that without faculty training, the quality of MCQs is generally poor. However, with faculty training the quality of MCQ can be very significantly improved.)

HATALA, R. & NORMAN, G.R. (2002) Adapting key feature examination for a clinical clerkship, *Med. Edu.* **36**: 160–165.

(An experiment with small-scale implementation of KF shows that a reasonable degree of generalizability can be achieved with small numbers of KF items.)

HIJAZI, Z., PREMADASA, I.G., & MOUSSA, M.A.A.A. (2002) Performance of students in the final examination in paediatrics: importance of short cases, *Arch. Dis. Childhood* **86**: 57–58.

HOLMBOE, E.S., HUOT, S., CHUNG, J., NORCINI, J., & HAWKINS, R.E. (2003) Construct validity of the miniclinical evaluation exercise (mini-CEX), *Acad. Med.* **78**(8): 826–830. Web address: http://www.academicmedicine.org/cgi/content/full/78/8/826.

(A research article validating mini-CEX.)

*HOLMBOE, E.S., HAWKINS, R.E., & HUOT, S.J. (2004) Effects of training in direct observation of medical residents' clinical competence: a randomized trial, *Ann. Inter. Med.* **140**(11): 874–881. Web address: http://www.annals.org/cgi/reprint/140/11/874.pdf.

(A RCT showing the importance of faculty training in improving rating.)

KARUNATHILAKE, I. & DAVIS, M. (2005) The place of oral examination in today's assessment system, *Med. Teacher* **27**(4): 294–297.

KOGAN, J.R., BELLINI, L.M., & SHEA, J.A. (2002) Implementation of the mini-CEX to evaluate medical students' clinical skills, *Acad. Med.* 77(11): 1156–1157.

LIM, J., CHAN, N., & CHEONG, P. (1998) Experience with portfolio-based learning in family medicine for Master of Medicine Degree, *Sing. Med. J.* **39**: 543–546.

(A descriptive article on one-page-portfolio from Singapore.)

LONKA, K., SLOTTE, V., HALTTUNEN, K. T., TIITINEN, A., VAARA, L., PAAOVONEN, J. (2001) Portfolios as a learning tool in obstetrics and gynaecology undergraduate training, *Med. Edu.* **35**(12): 1125–1130.

*LYNCH, D.C. & SWING, S.R. (2005) Key considerations for selecting assessment instruments and implementing assessment systems. ACGME. Web address: http://www.acgme.org/outcome/assess/keyConsider.asp.

(Part of the ACGME Outcome Project; a succinct discussion on factors that need to be considered in selecting assessment methods.)

MCGUIRE, C. (1999) George E Miller, MD, 1919–1998, *Med. Edu.* **33**: 312–314.

(An obituary on Prof George Miller; describes the early work of this pioneer in medical education. Fascinating read.)

**MEDICAL COUNCIL OF CANADA. Objectives for the qualifying examination, 3rd ed. http://www.mcc.ca/Objectives_online/

(A very well developed set of objectives listed under presenting problems. Easily browseable and freely available.)

MILLER, G.E. (1990) The assessment of clinical skills/competence/performance, *Acad. Med.* **65**(9): S63–S67.

MODERNISING MEDICAL CAREER. Direct Observation of Procedural Skills. National Health Service. Web address: http://www.mmc.nhs.uk/pages/assessment/dops.

MODERNISING MEDICAL CAREER. Mini-CEX (Clinical Evaluation Exercise), National Health Service. Web address: http://www.mmc.nhs.uk/pages/assessment/minicex.

MODERNISING MEDICAL CAREER. Multi-source feedback, National Health Service. Web address: http://www.mmc.nhs.uk/pages/assessment/msf.

MRCP (UK) — The clinical examination: practical assessment of clinical examination skills. Web address: http://www.mrcpuk.org/plain/PACES.html.

NEWBLE, D. & SWANSON, D.B. (1988) Psychometric characteristics of the objective structured clinical test, *Med. Edu.* **22**(4): 325–334.

*NEWBLE, D. (1998) Assessment. In: *Medical Education in the Millennium*, Jolly B and Rees L (eds.), 131–142 (Oxford University Press, Oxford, UK).

(Highly recommended reading for those who want to learn more about contemporary medical education.)

NORCINI, J.J., BLANK, L.L., DUFFY, F.D., & FORTNA, G.S. (2003) The mini-CEX: a method for assessing clinical skills, *Ann. Inter. Med.* **138**(6): 476–481. Web address: http://www.annals.org/cgi/reprint/138/6/476.

*NORCINI, J.J. (2003) Setting standard on educational test, *Med. Edu.* **37**: 464–469.

(A practical guide on standard setting. Recommended.)

NORCINI, J.J., BLANK, L.L., ARNOLD, G.K., & KIMBALL, H.R. (1995) Mini-CEX (Clinical Evaluation Exercise) a preliminary investigation, *Ann. Inter. Med.* **123**(10): 795–799. Web address: http://www.annals.org/cgi/content/full/123/10/795.

NORCINI, J.J. (2002) The death of the long case? *BMJ* **324: 408–409. Web address: http://www.pubmedcentral.nih.gov/articlerender.fcgi?artid=65539.

(In two pages, Dr Norcini provides a powerful argument against using long cases during examination. Include eye-opening psychometric values of many assessment instruments that we use commonly. Must read.)

*NORCINI J.J., DISERENS, D., DAY, S.C., *et al.* (1990) The scoring and reproducibility of an essay test of clinical judgment, *Acad. Med.* **65**(9): S41–S42.

(Research undertaken by the ABIM to determine the reliability and generalizability of long essay question.)

NORCINI, J.J., SWANSON, D.B., GROSSO, L.J., & WEBSTER, G.D. (1985) Reliability, validity and efficiency of multiple choice question and patient management problem item formats in assessment of clinical competence, *Med. Edu.* **19**(3): 238–247.

NØRGAARD, K., RINGSTED, C., & DOLMANS, D. (2004) Validation of a checklist to assess ward round performance in internal medicine, *Med. Edu.* **38**: 700–707.

NORMAN, G. (2003) Post graduate assessment – reliability and validity, *Trans. J. Coll. Med. S. Afri.* **47: 71–75.

(A highly readable text that discusses the implications of the Generalizability theory and case specificity in the selection of assessment instrument. Highly recommended.)

*PAGE, G. & BORDAGE, G. (1995) The Medical Council of Canada's key feature project: a more valid written examination of clinical decision making skills, *Acad. Med.* **70**(2): 104–110.

*PAGE, G., BORDAGE, G., & ALLEN, T. (1995) Developing key-feature problem and examination to assess clinical decision making skills, *Acad. Med.* **70**(3): 194–201.

(Describes comprehensive data from the development and evaluation phase of the key feature project.)

*PELLEGRINO, J.W., CHUDOWSKY N., & GLASSER R. (2001) Editors. Contribution of measurement and statistical modelling of assessment. In: *Knowing What Students Know: The Science and Design of Educational Assessment* (National Academy Press, Washington, DC, USA).

(Comprehensive coverage of assessment from a very reputable organization.)

RADEMAKERS, J., ten CATE, TH. J., & BÄR, P.R. (2005) Progress testing with short answer questions, *Med. Teacher* **27**(7): 578–582.

RAKSHA, J., LING, F.W., & JAEGER, J. (2004) Assessment of a 360-degree instrument to evaluate residents' competency in interpersonal and communication skills, *Acad. Med.* **79**: 458–463.

RUDNER, L.M-S. & WILLIAM, D. (2001) Reliability, *ERIC Digest*. ERIC Identifier: ED458213; Web address: http://www.ericdigests.org/2002-2/reliability.htm.

*SCHUWIRTH, L.W.T. & VLEUTEN, van der C.P.M. (2003) Written assessment. In: Cantillon P, Huthchison L, Wood D (eds.), *ABC of Learning and Teaching in Medicine* (BMJ Publishing Group, UK).

(A highly readable series of articles that covers topics that are needed by a medical teacher. Individual articles are available from BMJ's website.)

SCHUWIRTH, L.W.T. & VLEUTEN, van der C.P.M. (2004) Changing education, changing assessment, changing research? *Med. Edu.* **38**(8): 805–812.

SHEPARD, E. & GODWIN, J. (2004) Assessments through the learning process, *Question mark White Paper*, Questionmark Corporation. Web address: http://questionmark.com/us/home.htm.

*SMEE, S. (2003) Skill based assessment, *BMJ* **326**: 703–706. Web address: http://bmj.bmjjournals.com/cgi/reprint/326/7391/703.

(Simple reading. Recommended.)

SWANSON, D.B. (1987) A measurement framework for performance based test. In: Hart I.R., Harden, R.M. (eds.), *Further Developments in Assessing Clinical Competence*. Montreal Can–Heal.

TURNBULL, J., MACFADYEN, J., BARNEVELD, C. VAN, & NORMAN, G. (2000) Clinical work sampling: a new approach to the problem of in-training evaluation, *J. Gen. Inter. Med.* **15**: 556–561.

WASS, V., VLEUTEN, van der C.P.M., SHATZER, J., & JONES, R. (2001) Assessment of clinical competence, *The Lancet* **357: 945–949.

(A powerful article on the various methods of student assessment. Argues convincingly for the need for multiple samplings. Highly recommended.)

VLEUTEN, van der C.P.M. (2000) Validity of final examination in undergraduate medical training, *BMJ* **321**: 1217–1219.

WASS, V., JONES, R. & VLEUTEN, van der C.P.M. (2001) Standardized or real patients to test clinical competence? The long case revisited, *Med. Edu.* **35**: 321–325.

*WASS, V., VLEUTEN van der C., SHATZER, J., & JONES, R. (2001) Assessment of clinical competence, *The Lancet* **357**: 945–949.

WAUGH, D. & MOYSE, C.A. (1969) Oral examination: a videotape study of the reproducibility of grades in pathology, *Can. Med. Assoc. J.* **100**: 635–640.

WOJTCZAK, A. (2002) Glossary of medical education terms. Institute of International Medical Education (IIME). Web address: http://www.iime.org/glossary.htm#C

(Detailed listing of medical education terms.)

Index

About the Authors

Dr Zubair Amin is a pediatrician and medical educator. He was trained in Pediatrics in the University of Illinoise at Chicago. He has a Master in Health Profession Education (MHPE) from the same university. His interests and expertise are in assessment, staff development and international medical education.

Dr Chong Yap Seng is an obstetrician and educational leader. He is a graduate from National University of Singapore. He is deeply involved in undergraduate and post-graduate education, faculty training, assessment and scientific writing. He is the Head of Medical Education Unit, Yong Loo Lin School of Medicine.

Dr Khoo Hoon Eng is Associate Professor in the Dept of Biochemistry, Yong Loo Lin School of Medicine, National University of Singapore. She has a BA from Smith College, USA, PhD from University of London and Diploma in Medical Education from University of Dundee, UK. Her interests are in PBL, faculty training, and assessment.